The Fighter's Body
An Owner's Manual

The Fighter's Body

An Owner's Manual

*Your Guide to Diet, Nutrition, Exercise and Excellence
in the Martial Arts*

Loren W. Christensen   Wim Demerre

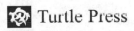 Turtle Press   Hartford

To contact the author or to order additional copies of this book:

   Turtle Press
   P.O. Box 290206
   Wethersfield, CT 06129-0206
   1-800-778-8785
   www.turtlepress.com

ISBN 1-880336-81-2

LCCN 2003011969

Printed in the United States of America

10 9

Library of Congress Cataloging-in-Publication Data

Christensen, Loren W.
  The fighter's body : an owner's manual your guide to diet, nutrition, exercise, and excellence in the martial arts / by Loren W. Christensen and Wim Demeere.
       p. cm.
Includes bibliographical references and index.
  ISBN 1-880336-81-2 (trade paper)
  1. Martial arts—Health aspects. 2. Martial artists—Nutrition. 3. Physical fitness. I. Demeere, Wim. II. Title.
  RC1220.M36 C48 2003
   613.7'148—dc21   2003011969

Contents

Acknowledgements

*To my three fantastic children, Carrie, Dan and Amy, who
are always supportive of my writing projects*
— Dad/Loren Christensen

To Nadja Talpaert, for her endless support and patience
— Wim Demeere

Many thanks to the photographers:

Donna Christensen
Gert Morren
Nadja Talpaert
Carsten Turf

Special thanks to our patient models:

Anneke Bosmans
Amy Christensen
Dan Christensen
Donna Duff-Christensen
Wim Willems

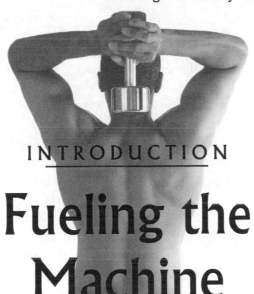

INTRODUCTION

Fueling the Machine

Most bodybuilders agree that proper nutrition is 60 percent of their effort in building the healthiest, strongest and most visually appealing physique possible. Pick up any magazine on running and at least a third if not half of the articles discuss how carbohydrates, fats, proteins, calories, water, vitamins and minerals all play a vital role in helping the runner progress in speed, explosiveness, endurance, and to recuperate quickly to run again the next day. Top swimmers certainly understand the importance of super nutrition, as do skaters, skiers, gymnasts, track and field athletes, power lifters and wrestlers.

More and more martial artists are now learning what top athletes in other sport activities have known for a long while: You don't put cheap, low-grade fuel in a high-performance car. If off track you want to run as smoothly as a BMW and on track you want to roar like an 800-horsepower Nascar at over 200 MPH,

you must put high-performance fuel in your tank.

Too many martial artists — whether they train in kung fu, karate, judo, tai chi, jujitsu, taekwondo, aikido, or the myriad of other great martial arts systems — rarely give a second thought as to how they fuel their bodies before or after their training or competition, nor do they consider how a healthy lifestyle fits into their fighting performance and progress. But those who are discovering the vital importance of eating well, getting sufficient sleep and training to build rather than tear down are discovering happily and enthusiastically that they feel better, look better and are improving in their fighting art faster than at any other time.

As a martial artist, you are cut from a different mold. You train in a unique activity in which you do battle with others and do battle with yourself. You sweat and strain, kick and punch, grapple and fall, dab blood from your lip and rub hurt muscles — and you pay dues to do these things! Is there something wrong with you? No. In fact, there is something wonderfully right about you. You are a unique individual. You are a warrior. While others flee the battle, you train for it in an environment that encourages you to get better and better at it.

While the fighting arts have been in existence since the first caveman whacked another caveman with the jawbone of a dinosaur, it has only been in recent years that modern fighters have discovered the power of nutrition and other healthy lifestyle choices to enhance their development. In some cases, "enhance" is an insufficient word as some fighters report that their progress has skyrocketed, while their injury and illness rate has been halved.

That is the good news. Now here is the really good news: It's not hard to do. It's not rocket science and it doesn't cost you an arm and a leg. All it takes is discipline, that same tough discipline that gets you to the training hall every workout day.

The Fighter's Body: An Owner's Manual is much more than a book about how you can get a flat, hard stomach. While there is something to be said for pleasing physical aesthetics, the real purpose of your authors' effort is show you how to use food, supplements, vitamins, minerals, and fluids to have better workouts, compete at your best, lose, maintain or increase your weight, and to ultimately walk down the mean streets with confidence knowing that

you are fit and raring to go should some hapless mugger make the grave mistake of picking on you. This book isn't about how to backfist faster or sidekick higher, but by learning how to fuel your body as if it were a high-performance race car, and by learning how to employ result-producing training regimens and rest and relaxation, all aspects of your martial arts will dramatically improve, and do so seemingly overnight.

Your authors have been there and done that. Wim Demeere began training in the martial arts as a teenager and over the years has studied a variety of fighting systems that have helped him come out on top in the mean streets and bring home the gold in grueling full-contact fighting events in his native country of Belgium and throughout the world. As a personal trainer, he teaches, trains and advises clients on health, exercise and the fighting arts.

Loren W. Christensen began training in karate and jujitsu in 1965 at the age of 19. Over the years he has used his skills to win over 50 tournaments and to survive deadly confrontations as a military policeman in Saigon, Vietnam and as a police officer for 25 years in Portland, Oregon. He has written and taught extensively on health, bodybuilding and the martial arts.

More important than our physical achievements is our on-going scholarly study of nutrition, supplementation, aerobic training, and the mental discipline needed to bring out the very best of which one is capable.

We don't believe in quick fixes because they don't work in the long run. Most are unhealthy, some are even detrimental and almost all are impossible to maintain. And we provide several examples and anecdotes to prove this. Instead, we believe in long-term, lifestyle fixes, and we believe in them for one simple reason: they work.

You will happily find that we aren't rigid drill sergeants. For instance, once we get the concept of a healthy life plan ingrained into your mind, we show you how to cheat a little and get away with it. How cool is that? (We so desperately want you to like us.)

Here are just some of the topics covered in these pages:

- **Need to drop a few pounds?** Follow these proven ways to trim it off and keep it off so you get more out of your training, improve your appearance and enjoy greater health.

- **Are you already in shape?** Learn how to stay that way as you get older.

- **Are you underweight?** Learn proven ways to combine eating, supplementation and exercise to put on muscle that adds awesome power to your punches, kicks and grappling.

- **Want to lose five or 10 pounds quickly?** Learn the best way to do it safely.

- **Want to stay in your weight division** or move up or down one? It's easy with these proven methods.

- **Confused about carbohydrates and protein grams?** Use these easy-to-follow formulas for determining how many you need for maximum energy and optimum muscle repair.

- **Are you drinking enough liquids?** Learn how water, sports drinks and even coffee can make you faster, stronger, and more energetic.

- **Want a hamburger?** Learn how to eat healthily at fast food joints.

- **Want a beer?** Find out how you can work a frosty one into your healthy lifestyle.

- **Want ice cream, cake and pizza?** Find out how to eat those goodies and still kick and punch like a real warrior.

- **Not sure if you can do it?** Oh, yes you can, and you will learn how to develop the right mind-set. The warrior mind.

We aren't going to lie to you like they do in some of those ads that claim you can drop 10 pounds in a week and develop a six-pack of stomach muscles in only three minutes a day. We do tell you how to achieve those goals, but know that it takes effort, discipline and more time than what the ads want you to believe. We don't baby you and tell you everything a lazy person wants to hear. But you can count on us for the truth and for information that is healthy and productive.

While nutrition is a complex field, we have made every effort to make it easy to understand. Once your mind is ready, we think you will find it a pleasant journey, one that has two destinations: a place where you enjoy greater health and a place where you achieve the best that you can be in your fighting art.

As students of health, diet, nutrition, exercise, psychology, personal motivation, and the martial arts, we know first hand that this information works because we have been proving it for over 55 combined years of training, teaching, coaching, advising and personal consultation. You won't find in these pages any of those whiz-bang, new supplements and diets that come out virtually every week. We present only that information that has proven itself over the years to have lasting results.

While this book could have been over a thousand pages of complex, boring data, we have worked hard to make the information succinct, usable and even fun. We have personally used every workout and eating plan presented here and, to make your path a smooth one, we have moved aside most of the obstacles and point out where others are hiding and waiting to spring like evil ninjas.

So, stir yourself up a protein shake and let's get started.

All things be ready if our minds be so
Henry V

Fast Facts

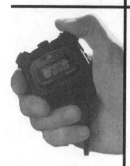

- The most common belief, one based on a whole lot of wishful thinking, is that crunches, hundreds of them, trim fat from the waistline.

- Crunches will develop strong abs for the power you need for your martial art techniques, but if you want them to show, you have to reduce your body fat.

- *Myth:* Eating after 8 PM makes you gain weight.

  Truth: Calories are the same at any hour of the day. However, eating at night tends to lead to consuming more calories than you need because you are home near the refrigerator and near the television where you are bombarded with commercials for high-calorie foods.

- Infomercials that push exercise and nutrition products zap us with, "See results in 10 days!" and "Get a defined midsection in less than three minutes a day!" While this does have a certain appeal, it unfortunately isn't the way the human body works.

- Basic, nutrition-rich foods, such as vegetables, fruit, and lean cuts of meat, are almost always cheaper than ready-made meals and dining out.

- Cutting calories drastically affects your metabolism; specifically, it slows it down, and the slower it goes the more likely you are to store fat.

- Do such labels as "health food," "natural" and "all natural" mean they are safe to use? Not necessarily.

- Maintaining your weight or dropping a few pounds needs to be approached from all angles; eating low-fat foods is just one.

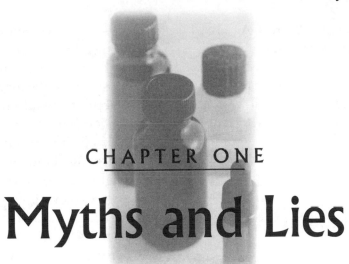

CHAPTER ONE

Myths and Lies

Co-author Christensen recalls hearing the following conversation in a health club between a pumped, steroid-sopped bodybuilder and an easily swayed 24-year-old just beginning to lift weights.

Pumped bodybuilder: "Hey man. You wanna buy some 'roids? Guaranteed to get you big."

Skinny guy: "Oh no, sir. My wife and I are trying to have a child and I don't want it to be born with problems 'cause I took steroids."

Pumped bodybuilder: "That won't happen, man."

Skinny guy: "It won't? Oh, okay. How much are they?"

That is all the convincing it took to get this beginner to change his mind and buy an unknown, toxic substance to put into his body. He didn't research it or talk to a health professional; he simply made a snap decision about something

that would affect his entire body, inside and out, based on what a gym rat told him. Why? Because he wanted it to be true.

Myths exist year after year because so many people want to believe in them. We are not just talking about those people who are convinced there are trolls living under bridges or people who believe they are routinely whisked away to other planets. We are talking about mature, educated and worldly people - teachers, lawyers, nurses, judges, and athletes, including martial artists - who want to believe that there is an easy, sweatless and quick way to get healthy, strong, lean, hairless, and get blindingly white teeth.

Let's narrow it down and look at some of the many myths surrounding the not-so-exact-science of high-powered nutrition, exercise and weight loss. Few of these go away because so many want so desperately to believe they are true. Remember, if it sounds too good to be true, well, you know the rest. As a hard training martial artist, you put tremendous demand on your body. To have healthy longevity in the fighting arts, knowledge is critical as to which methods are likely to work, which are dangerous and which wastes your time.

Spot Reduction

Just when we think the concept of spot reduction has gone away, it returns to lead folks down the path of wasted effort. The false belief is this: Work a specific muscle or muscle group especially hard and fat just melts away from that very spot.

The most common belief, one based on a whole lot of wishful thinking, is that crunches, hundreds of them, trim fat from the waistline. Convincing you that this is possible puts money in the pockets of swindlers who every six months come out with a new abdominal contraption that promises on their grandmothers' graves to not only melt away abdominal muck, but do so in - say it with us - only three minutes a day. If that wasn't enough, the commercials suggest that in the end, an attractive and admiring hot babe or stud will hang off your arm and gaze longingly into your eyes. Unfortunately, it doesn't work that way. Hey, don't kill the messengers.

Where you accumulate fat depends on numerous factors: genetic make up (blame your parents), gender (men usually store more around their

stomachs, while women store more around their hips), your activities, and many others. Making your life even more miserable is the tendency for your body to burn fat first from where it last packed it on. For example, if you accumulated it first around your midsection, that is going to be the last and toughest place for you to trim. Those places on your body with the least fat will be the first to show the visible effects from calorie reduction and increased calorie burning from exercise. Sometimes this might be exactly what you want, while other times it might lead to a disproportionate esthetic effect (a fancy way of saying you look funny in the nude).

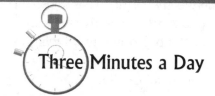

Three Minutes a Day

The claim "in just three minutes a day" is used in many magazine ads and infomercials because it sells products. Technically, you will lose a little fat in three minutes, but the loss is so microscopic that you should be able to fit into your new training pants in, oh, about three years. Here is why.

A 170-pound person jogging for three minutes burns about 35 calories, about what is in half a small chocolate chip cookie. Do the math and you find that this person has to jog 100 three-minute sessions to lose 3,500 calories, the amount in one pound of fat. Since ab crunches don't burn as many calories as jogging, it's going to take you a long, long while to reach your goal.

Without a sensible eating plan, doing crunches until you drip blood from your belly button won't give you that coveted washboard abdominal region as long as there is a layer of fat covering it. Crunches will develop strong abs for the power you need for your martial art techniques, but if you want them to show, you have to reduce your body fat. Now, if you just reduce fat without developing a muscular midsection, you will just look skinny. But when you follow a good ab program and diet that coveted ripped look will be yours. So, before you do your next set of 500-rep crunches to burn off fat, think about this bumper sticker.

Abs are made in the gym and in the kitchen

We aren't going to tell you that reducing fat and developing a strong midsection is easy, because it's not. On the other hand, it's not terribly difficult either. It just takes knowledge and discipline. In subsequent chapters we show you how sound dietary habits and exercises aimed at your entire body stimulate overall weight loss, including ridding the midsection of fat. We even show you how to get maximum benefit out of just a few crunches. Before you get giddy, though, know that these crunches are tough and make the veins in your forehead stick out. But you can do it.

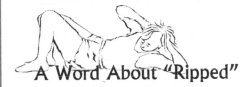

A Word About "Ripped"

A ripped midsection isn't mandatory for optimum martial arts performance. Case in point: Movie star/martial artist Samo Hung, star of *Martial Law* and numerous kung fu movies, moves extremely well for an overweight fighter. But he is a rare exception, as few martial artists carrying extra pounds move with such grace and speed. We use the term ripped and its visual image as a way of describing an ideal, one that affords you strength for your techniques and one that offers visual proof of your conditioning.

If you are currently soft around the middle, but four months from now you have developed a six-pack of ab muscles as a result of discipline at the dinner table and in your training, feel proud of your accomplishment. However, if you choose not to reduce your body fat to the extent that your developed abs show (some people naturally have a thin layer of fat over their abdomen), it's okay as long as they are strong.

I'll Just Eat Less to Lose Weight

The assumption with this myth is this: Eating makes me fat. Therefore, I'll eat less and I won't get fat. People who cut calories radically or skip meals "to drop a couple of pounds" are following the assumption to its seemingly logical conclusion.

Sorry, it doesn't work that way. In actuality, cutting calories drastically affects your metabolism; specifically, it slows it down, and the slower it goes the more likely you are to store fat. Yes, store it. It's a cruel joke: eat a whole lot less, and get fat. Real funny!

Stress Reactions to Excessive Calorie Reduction

The human body knows two powerful stress reactions: Acute and prolonged. Think of acute stress as how you react physiologically when a mugger jumps out from the dark and points a knife at your face: Your body dumps adrenaline instantly into your system for fight or flight. Think of prolonged stress as the physiological reaction of being trapped in a collapsed house for several days after an earthquake without food and water: To survive, your metabolism slows down and energy drains from your muscles, digestive system and sexual system, using it mostly for primary functions, such as thinking, breathing and keeping your heart beating. Your system becomes highly efficient with its resources when it figures out that it's not getting the usual amount of nourishment it needs.

This is a survival mechanism (probably left over from our caveman days) that keeps you alive when food is at a minimum. So when you skip meals and drastically cut calories, your body can't differentiate between a real famine and you just deciding not to eat. It just knows it's starving, and slows down your metabolism to desperately hold on to every critical calorie it gets. It's a fight your body wins, which means those love handles are going to cling fast to your sides.

Here is more bad news: The fact that you are always hungry ultimately leads to binging and overeating, and when that happens, your body thinks, "Finally, some food! I'd better store it for later," and retains as many calories as possible as — you guessed it — icky fat. Dr. Catherine Steiner-Adair, director of education, prevention, and outreach at the Harvard Eating Disorders Center (a division of Harvard Medical School) who treats eating disorders says, "If you begin to restrict or think obesssively about food, you are very likely to binge."[1]

You can gain weight due to the famine stress reaction, even when eating only twice a day and with limited portions. Consider this incredible story. A woman complained to her doctor about being depressed and having low energy. When asked what she ate, she told him she had one bowl of soup at lunch and one yogurt at dinner. That was it. Nothing else. Not even a raisin. Since she wasn't consuming enough calories in those two "meals" to sustain her basic dietary needs, she was constantly fatigued and depressed. On weekends, she rewarded herself for all her suffering by binging on junk food, which accounted for her overweight condition. This is because her body frantically accumulated all the calories in her fat cells to use as energy during the long week of starvation. She had been following the I'll-just-eat-less-and-lose-weight logic for five years, never once questioning that it just might be the root of her problems. Her doctor immediately saw what was happening and put her on a healthy diet with fixed times to eat throughout the day. Within one week, she dropped three pounds and immediately began to enjoy greater energy and a happier outlook.

Lack of Energy

This will be discussed in detail later, but for now know that you cannot get a productive workout when skipping meals and cutting calories drastically. Calories are not bad guys; you need them desperately to train, compete, strategize, and recuperate. Later we provide you with several plans to cut calories intelligently so you can still slam and bam with energy to spare.

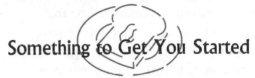

Something to Get You Started

Later, we give you several ways to reduce calories, but here is a trick you can start using right now since it's used in all of our eating plans: Eat frequent, small meals throughout the day. This prevents your body from declaring a famine and defensively retaining all the calories and nutrients it can get. By eating five or six small meals throughout your waking hours, you speed up your metabolism, which sends your body the opposite signal: It has enough calories and nutrients for what lies ahead.

One other benefit, which sounds almost too good to be true, is that since it takes a lot of calories to digest your food, eating several meals a day turns your body into an efficient calorie-burning machine. In other words, the more often you eat the more calories you burn. Life doesn't get much better than that. Additionally, you enjoy ample and consistent energy from the moment you get up until you crash into your bed 16 hours later. More on frequent meals in subsequent chapters.

I'll Stop Eating Fat to Lose Weight

We don't state many absolutes in this book because it's difficult to do so when discussing how the human body reacts to various programs. That said, here is one absolute about dieting, or more specifically, about calories. As you know, there are gazillions (read: a lot) of diets in books, magazines, on the internet and on photocopies passed around the office. Some are good, some are absurd (the beer and steak diet comes to mind. Darn it!), and others are seriously dangerous to your health. There are diets designed around eating only vegetables, eating only meat and a popular one at this writing that touts the wonders of eating lots of fat.

If any of these diets work, whether they are the healthy ones or the crazy ones, it's because of one reason and one reason only: Your body uses more calories in its daily activities than it takes in. It doesn't care if the calories are from fat, carbohydrates (carbs) or protein. If you eat fewer than what your body needs to train, work, play, sleep or zone out in front of the tube, you lose weight. It's a simple concept. There is no argument.

Since fat holds more calories than carbs and protein, it would seem that fat is the bad guy in your diet. Much of this myth comes from the negative connotation conveyed by the word. We want to trim fat from our waistlines; our butt is too fat, our thighs are too fat. Therefore, fat is bad. While that seems logical, it's dangerously incorrect.

The truth is that there are vital biochemical functions in your body that need fat. For example, fat is required to maintain a correct hormonal balance, maintain healthy skin, maintain a healthy testosterone level, and absorb certain vitamins. Totally eliminating it would lead to illness. Even if it were possible for you to avoid dietary fat altogether, you wouldn't lose weight if you consumed more protein and carb calories than you use in your daily activities.

Make fat a part of your diet, just make sure it's not the biggest part. More on fat in Chapters 3 and 4.

Why You Crave Fat

Fat cells supply you with energy and protect you from hunger and cold. Eating it is a primal survival mechanism you inherited from your prehistoric ancestors. In their era, fat was a valuable commodity, but in your world, it's ever-present. Unfortunately, the survival mechanism still works to make you crave the stuff. Eliminate or drastically reduce it, and you soon hunger for it, and hunger desperately as it gives texture, flavor and taste to food. You become obsessed, especially for burgers, chips, milkshakes, cupcakes, and other high-fat goodies. When you do give in, usually after rationalizing that you need it, you overindulge.

It's More Expensive to Eat Healthily

This is patently untrue. Basic, nutrition-rich foods, such as vegetables, fruit and lean cuts of meat, are almost always cheaper than ready-made meals and dining out. Take advantage of the time of year and buy whatever fruit and vegetables are in season and at their lowest price. Get to know the stores in your community, since one might offer the best buy for fresh foods and another the best buy for lean cuts of meat.

Want a snack? A medium-sized, 100-calorie apple with no fat costs you about 50 cents, while a chocolate bar, a 300 calorie, fat laden chocolate bar, costs about a dollar. If you don't know which of those are the best for your kicking and punching body, you soon will as you delve deeper into these pages.

Eating After 8 PM Makes You Fat

This myth is based on the fact that since you don't use many calories after 8 PM, any you take in are stored as body fat. Maybe they will, maybe they won't. Once again, it's all about calories; in this case, it's about how many you consume before 8 PM. Let's say you need 2000 calories a day to maintain your weight, and today at breakfast, at your midmorning snack and at lunch, you took in a total of 1,300. This means at your afternoon snack and at dinner, you can have no more than 700 calories.

That's it. You are done eating for the day. If you do have a little something beyond your 2000, say, 300 calories worth of something, there is a good chance it will accumulate as fat. The solution, therefore, is to take in 1,800 in your fist five meals, so that you can have 200 calories for an evening snack.

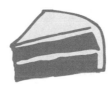

How It Typically Happens

You just had a grueling, seemingly endless day at school or work, and then you raced across town to your martial arts school, trained to exhaustion, and then raced back across town to your home, where you collapsed onto your sofa in a heap of fatigue and stress. It's 8:30. After you catch your breath, you have one simple thought: chips and a comfort drink, pop or beer. Since you haven't had your evening meal, you rationalize that your fatigue and stress entitles you to pork out and, what the heck, enjoy a second comfort drink.

If all this comfort eating takes place after you have eaten your 2000 calories, you are on your way to Fatville City, but only because you ate more than 2000, not because you gorged it down after 8 PM. Later we discuss the harm such junk food does to your body after a hard workout.

Don't allow stress, fatigue, and need for comfort to be an excuse to overeat, whether it's healthy food or high-fat junk. Don't listen to that syrupy, evil voice of rationalization: "Come on. You trained like a crazy person. You earned a triple burger and milkshake. And some fudge. 'Cause you're a killer." You must resist, and resist hard because fatigue and stress can weaken your willpower. Use your discipline, the same discipline you use to go to your martial arts school on hot summer days and do 200 punches and 200 kicks when your friends are sitting in the shade at the park. If you do weaken and yield to The Evil Voice, your evening will end with hundreds of excess calories hanging off your gut. Think of them as designer calories, designed to make your belly larger.

Bottom line: If by bedtime you have taken in more calories than you used during the day, you get a glob of fat somewhere on your body. To phrase this more positively: It doesn't matter when you eat during a 24-hour period, as long as you eat only the calories you need. Do that and you will be a lean, mean fighting machine.

Free tip 1: Dinner is often the only hot meal eaten by people with fast-paced lives, food that frequently contains calorie monsters like gravy, casseroles and so on. Know that cold foods often contain fewer calories.

Free tip 2: Here is an idea that works for some fighters. Plan your daily meals in such a way that your martial arts workout follows the meal with the most calories. You have to have enough energy to train anyway, so combine a big meal (not too big) with a hard training session that burns lots of calories.

Natural or Herbal Weight-loss Products Are Safe and Effective

Over the last decade there has been a veritable boon of interest in so-called "natural" products, a movement that is hardly surprising considering the industrialization of the food industry. What we get today on our plate has never been more altered, enriched, colored, processed, tweaked, massaged (in Japan they actually massage cows to improve the meat), and who knows what else. Check out the labels and you find conserving agents, taste enhancers, color additives and all kinds of unpronounceable chemicals.

Scary fact: Many of the same chemicals added to your food are also found in cleaning agents, dyes and a host of other products found under your sink.

As interest in health, nutrition and exercise has increased over the years, enlightened consumers are more aware now of the low nutritional value and health risks in many ingredients added to packaged foods. Due to the growing interest in natural foods, virtually every major supermarket today has a "health" section where you can find food products that have not been sprayed, colored or supplemented with chemicals. In the same aisle are rows of herbal products that fall under the same "all natural" label.

So do such labels as "health food," "natural" and "all natural" mean they are safe to use? Not necessarily. Always keep in mind that many companies selling these products are just as motivated to relieve you of your money as are the infomercial people (discussed in a moment), and are often just as quick with half-truths, unsubstantiated claims and just plain verbal rubbish. Yes, some of these products are good for you, but others have no value whatsoever, and those remaining might be downright dangerous. Due to the litigious society we now live in, many companies have started to cover themselves by adding large disclaimers on their products.

We found one product that has the following script on its label: "The dietary supplement [X] consists of only the finest natural herbs gathered from over 12 countries of the world. All our products are manufactured in the United States at our government-inspected facilities. We are a leader in quality with every product meeting the highest standards of the industry." Written by the product's marketing people, these sentences are designed to put your mind at ease as to the product's safety and effectiveness. You read it and conclude that the product is natural and safe. Maybe it is, but just below the script are these bold-capped words: **"READ ENTIRE LABEL**

WARNING IMMEDIATELY BELOW." The text that follows, also in caps, warns you against using the product if pregnant, if you have a history or a family history of heart or thyroid disease, diabetes, high blood pressure, recurrent headaches, depression, any psychiatric condition, glaucoma, difficulty urinating, enlarged prostate, and many other medical conditions. Buried deeply in the warning is a further warning that you might experience "serious adverse health effects" if you take the product with caffeine. Surprisingly, people are still buying this, though there has to be a significant percentage who fall into one or more of the at-risk categories.

The question that needs to be asked is this: If an all-natural product is completely safe, why are there so many conditions that prohibit its use? Should all products labeled "natural" be considered unsafe? Well, we wouldn't go that far. But since it's not always easy to tell, it's best to never use them indiscriminately. Read the labels, adhere to the warnings, and when in doubt, contact your physician.

Don't be fooled by the flashy labeling on the products or the finely honed sales pitch from the slick-looking dude in the infomercial. Natural or herbal products aren't a sure bet. While some produce good results, many others aren't worth your hard-earned cash. Educate yourself about any product you put into your body. Research it and talk with your physician or dietitian. Then listen to that little voice of common sense in your head when strolling through the health section of your supermarket.

Low-fat Food is Healthier but Tastes Terrible

There is some truth to this, though "terrible" is in the taste buds of the, uh, chewer. A friend of Christensen's once shared a no-fat muffin with him as they drank coffee together. Christensen says it not only tasted horrible, but it had a consistency of chewing gum, and at one point it got caught half way down his throat. At first he tried to massage the outside of his neck to get it unstuck, then he went into a retching fit, looking a little like a cat with a fir ball in its throat.

As mentioned earlier, fat adds flavor to food and gives us a sense of feeling full. This doesn't necessarily mean that all low-fat food is devoid of flavor. Again, that is up to each person to decide. Christensen's friend chomped on the muffin with obvious pleasure, while Christensen prayed the man was adept at the Heimlich maneuver. The good news is that people in the food industry are working to develop more flavorful low-fat foods that taste closer to those that contain more fat.

Maintaining your weight or dropping a few pounds needs to be approached from all angles; eating low-fat foods is just one. If you try to survive solely on low- and no-fat foods, you soon will go mad and fling yourself from the roof of a high-rise building. To ensure this doesn't happen, eat only those low- and no-fat foods you like, while keeping an open mind to try others. Don't overindulge. They still contain calories, sometimes lots of them. For example,

two of those Volkswagen-sized muffins contain enough calories to keep a room of kindergartners looting and pilfering for hours. Eat low- and no-fat foods as part of your overall plan, but you still need to count the calories.

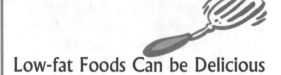

Low-fat Foods Can be Delicious

If you happen to be a kitchen warrior, know that with some creativity you can whip up a delicious low-fat meal that just might be tastier than those artery-choking, high-fat ones. There are zillions of low-fat cookbooks on the market and gazillions of low-fat recipes on the internet. Test it out on the net: Keyword "low-fat chicken and Spanish rice" into the search box of your favorite search engine. You get mucho recipes.

When one flavor dominates, it's often less enjoyable than meals that offer a variety of tastes. The flavors in many packaged foods, for example, are poorly balanced so that the dominant flavors - salt, barbeque sauce, cheese, hot sauce — prevent you from distinguishing subtle nuances. This can lead to overeating as you unconsciously search for a greater variety of tastes.

Make your meals flavor intense. The best recipes are those that give you balance in flavor and nutrition. Do a little research on cooking low-fat meals to see how you can combine different flavors to create a delicious meal without consuming volumes of calories.

Low-fat Foods are Best for Losing Weight

Along with herbal and natural products, low-fat foods have — as a result of clever marketing — taken the world by storm. Today, virtually every type of food on the market has a low-fat version. The smart marketers slap on appealing labels, such as "low-fat," "light," "fat-free" and "reduced-fat" and then charge more than their fat counterparts. However, all this creative verbiage about the product's fat content ignores or deliberately hides one important question: Exactly how low, how light, how free and how reduced is the fat in the product? Five percent? Ten? More? Less?

These are vague labels (deliberately so?) and their meaning varies from one product to the next. The food industry might have a mandate as to how foods are labeled, but it's still incredibly confusing to consumers. You might find a good tasting low-fat candy bar that contains only two-percent fat, while another brand, also displaying a low-fat label, contains a higher percentage. Not only might there be a difference between two low-fat candy bars, it could be a significant difference. This is why it's important that you always check the nutrition value table on all products. While the terms low, reduced and light are not consistent from product to product, the labeling laws are strict as to the quantity of carbs, fats, protein, calories, and micronutrients in the products.

Make special note of the calories in the low-fat products. Remember, your body doesn't care whether the excess calories came from carbs, protein or fat. Any unused calories get stored somewhere on your body. Know that low-fat, reduced-fat, and no-fat, doesn't necessarily mean low calories. Co-author Christensen learned this about three months after he discovered no-fat, frozen yogurt, sold in a quaint little shop a few blocks from his home. Since it had no fat, he naively assumed he could have an industrial-sized cone once a day, sometimes twice, sometimes dipped in chocolate. By the end of summer, his training uniform fit snugly and his martial arts moves had become sluggish, a result of about 15 pounds of unused calories — no-fat calories — surrounding his waistline.

One low-fat commercial cupcake, for instance, contains the same number of calories as a regular, high-fat cupcake, but because it's labeled low-fat it sells like, well, hotcakes. No doubt the naïve even eat two or three extra believing it's okay to do so. Learn from Christensen's discovery, the same sad one made by thousands of others, and don't overeat low-fat foods under the assumption that they contain fewer calories. Check the labels, check the labels, check the labels.

How They Still Get You

One reason why there aren't fewer calories in some low- or no-fat foods is that the manufacturers have added things to get you to eat them. Fat-free desserts, for example, often contain extra sugar, sometimes a lot of extra sugar, to compensate for the lack of rich taste lost when the fat was removed. What this means is the calories saved by eating a low- or no-fat desert come back to haunt, laugh and mock you in another form.

We aren't saying that you shouldn't eat these foods, but we are encouraging you to read the labels and keep your portions in check. Low- and no-fat products are a valuable addition to your diet, but they aren't a quick fix to losing weight. The manufacturers have spent a lot of money to fool consumers into believing that fat is the bad guy in your diet. While it's true that too much saturated fat can have detrimental effects on your health (we talk about this later), it's also true that eating too many calories, no matter where they come from, causes you to gain weight. This is a fact the admen haven't been able to change and almost always fail to mention.

Keep this fact in mind and hopefully it will help you remember to check the labels: *We now have more fat-free foods than ever before in history, but the population is growing ever more dangerously fat with each passing year.*

Don't let the ad men win. You are a warrior. Keep your guard up.

10 Diet Gimmicks to Ignore

By now you know that it's all about calories and anything you hear that claims otherwise, you should suspect immediately that they are evil, stinking low-life liars. That might be a little strong, but you get the point. Here are 10 diet cons that slim and trim — your bank account.

- **The program is effortless** Sure, and a kick in the groin is a lot of laughs. Losing weight takes time, effort and discipline. It's not always easy, but it's definitely worth the effort.

- **Your weight loss is permanent** Not if you resume eating and training the way you were before you began the diet. If after you lose the weight you maintain a sensible, calorie conscious eating plan and a good training regimen, the weight stays off. Eat more calories than you burn, however, and your old self comes back to strain your waistband.

- **Eat all the sausage and bacon you want** Even if this worked, do you really want to feed your heart and arteries all that fat? Along with a sensible reduction in calories, eat lots of fruit, veggies and lean meat to slim down healthily.

- **You need a Masters degree in chemistry to figure it out** This diet claims that you must eat only protein at one meal, carbs at the next and fat only on Sunday. Nonsense. There is no scientific proof that you can lose weight by not combining certain foods. It's okay; your body can handle bread and turkey at the same time.

- **Certain food groups are banned** Anytime you neglect a food group you risk suffering from a lack of nutrients. Your objective is to drop those unwanted pounds, but do so with lots of energy and with vibrant health.

- **They show before and after pictures of a guy who lost 50 pounds eating a brand name fast food** The more sensational the ad, the more you need to scrutinize the fine print. By law, the weight loss claimed from an advertised diet must be representative of all people, not just one person. If it's not, there must be a disclaimer that says something about the results not being typical.

- **You have to trace your ancestry** There are even wacko diets where you tailor your eating according to your blood type or where you eat similarly to your cave dwelling ancestors (this ignores the fact that few cavemen lived to see 30). Avoid these plans like a charging T-rex and spend your efforts on training hard and selecting healthy, low-cal foods.

- **Eat only watermelon and cheesecake** Hmm, this one sounds pretty good. But for six meals a day? While you might at first lose weight on a diet that allows you to eat only one or two types of food, such restriction is unhealthy because it lacks a variety of nutrients. Also, few people can remain on a diet that is so boring, and when they go off, it's — hello pizza.

- **Foods you have always known to be healthy are now bad for you** There are diets that claim nutrient-rich foods, such as beets, carrots and apples cause you to store excess sugar as fat. Nonsense. The only thing that causes you to store fat is too many unused calories.

- **You see it advertised at 2 AM on cable** Always keep in mind that the spokesperson's giddiness and dripping enthusiasm are part of an act. The pretty person is getting paid to get you excited over their wacky diet plan. Don't fall for it. Besides you should be sleeping, anyway.

Infomercials

Infomercials that push exercise and nutrition products zap us with, "See results in 10 days!" and "Get a defined midsection in less than three minutes a day!" While this does have a certain appeal, it unfortunately isn't the way the human body works. Now, some of the advertised products are indeed good, but the claims shouted by the ecstatic spokespersons are often laughable exaggerations of what is the truth. Actually, they aren't that funny when you think about how many hopeful people send in their hard-earned bucks for the stuff.

Anyone who has participated in physical training for at least a year knows that it takes time and effort to lose weight, to get aerobically fit and to develop the best body that genetics allow. While there are rare people who are genetically blessed and can achieve tremendous success faster than the rest of us (we so hate them), even they can't do it in 10 days, using three-minute workouts.

So why do people buy these infomercial products? Besides falling prey to the slick salesmanship, infomercials appeal to their desperate hope that there really is a magic bullet out there that gives results for little effort: larger breasts, whiter teeth, $10,000 a week working only two hours a day, rock hard abs, and self-defense skills from aerobic kickboxing. The con artists selling these hopes and dreams drive nice cars and wear flashy suits because people are buying, people who want to believe there is a shortcut to success, fame, health, and a youthful appearance. Even the word "infomercial" is a trap, as it suggests that what you are viewing isn't just a commercial but information, truthful information. More times than not, though, it's disinformation.

Over the many years that infomercials have been entertaining insomniacs and Sunday morning early risers, they have offered a host of products (besides spray-on hair and vibrating finger attachments) that promise an easy and fast path to a hard body: diet pills, abdominal exercisers and electrical muscle stimulating devices. While some products do give minimal results,

seldom are they sold with information that isn't distorted, exaggerated or falsified. Let's take a look at one product seen frequently on infomercials that has appealed to many martial artists.

Why They Can Lie to You

Have you ever torn your gaze from the attractive spokesperson and noticed the tiny print at the bottom of the screen that companies must display to cover themselves legally? The print usually reads like this.

"A sound diet is necessary for permanent weight loss."

"Individual results may vary."

With these barely visible phrases, the makers of infomercials are able to get away with twisting facts so that you buy their products. The fine print also prevents you from suing them when you sadly discover that you still have a big tummy though you followed their instructions and spent less than three minutes a day for 10 whole days on their goofy abdominal contraption.

Abdominal Machines

Setting aside the fact that some ab machines are bad for your back (co-author Christensen bought one of those) or that some do a terrible job of targeting the abdominal muscles, let's take a look at those oh-so-sincere claims made by those oh-so-attractive, bubbly spokespersons as to how they "burn calories" and award you with "a tight tummy and a sexy six-pack." Right, and cows fly in formation.

Here is a statement you will see many times in this book: To lose fat, you must burn more calories than you consume. Any physical activity you do beyond what is your normal daily activity burns extra calories. For example, should your TV remote suddenly die and you are forced to get up off your sofa 10 times in one evening to change channels (we pray that never happens to you), you will burn extra calories. Now, getting up and manually changing channels won't give you an awesome six pack of abs, but because it's an activity beyond what is normal for you, you will burn a few calories, roughly the same number contained in a couple of potato chips.

Likewise, since you normally don't exercise on that abdominal machine the partially clad spokesperson is pitching, doing so burns a few extra calories. Will that activity alone give you a defined midsection? Sorry, but no way. How about if you do it every day? Nope. You still have more work to do before you can show off your bellybutton ring.

Now, we aren't against all ab machines, per se; some are safe and some actually help you develop a strong midsection. However, it's our opinion that you really don't need an apparatus since there are hundreds of free-hand exercises that can be done without spending a dime. There are even martial art movements that work your abs (see Chapter 8). For now, just know that when you diet consistently and train intelligently, your six-pack will one day show itself in your bathroom mirror.

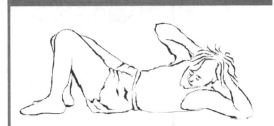

About 111,000 Reps Should Do It

To burn one lousy pound of body fat - 3,500 calories — on an ab machine, you would have to do thousands of reps, since it's an easy exercise and the abs are small compared to, say, the leg muscles. You would have to emulate a guy by the name of Edmar Freitas, a Brazilian weight-training instructor who cranked out 111,000 crunches in 24 hours for the Guinness World Records. If you choose to burn fat like ab-man Freitas, know that you are going to have to do it about every day, which means you have to scratch sleep, eating and going to the bathroom off your "Things-to-do-list."

Fast Facts

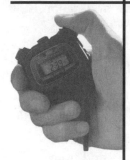

- Look at the diets of some well-known fighters and martial arts action stars, and it's amazing they can perform at all, let alone do well.

- You can't change the genes your parents gave you, but that doesn't mean you can't change your appearance to some degree.

- Ectomorphs generally have low body fat, small bones and very little muscle mass. Endomorphs have large bones, high body fat and not a lot of muscle mass. Mesomorphs have low to medium body fat levels and lots of muscle mass.

- When a genetically blessed fighter pushes his body through all the rigors of the martial arts but doesn't feed it the necessary macro and micronutrients, it's going to erode and even cannibalize itself for the nutrients it so desperately needs.

- Individuals react differently to carbs, protein and fat ratios. Know that just because a specific diet works for your karate teacher, doesn't mean that it will work for you, too.

- Since you can't see into the future, there is no way of knowing if an unhealthy habit, even a small one, will strike you down in your prime.

- We encourage you to read about champion fighters and movie martial artists, but never emulate them 100 percent, especially those anomalies who do everything considered bad for their health.

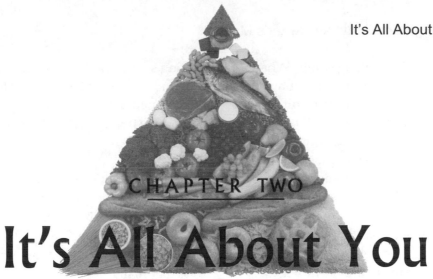

CHAPTER TWO

It's All About You

That Champion Eats Junk Food, Can You?

Sometimes martial arts masters, tournament champs and movie stars are regarded as nearly mythical. They throw head-high kicks seemingly without effort and at laser-like speed; their punches flail as fast as a mad drummer's sticks and, with today's movie technology, celluloid martial arts heroes can run up a wall, over the roof and down the other side. Many of these champions, whether real or reel, are placed on pedestals where every word they utter is taken as gospel. But with some of them, their words are not always wise. While their martial arts skill, publicity agents, magazine editors, tournament sponsors, and onscreen charisma have helped make them a household name in the martial arts world, they remain human, and as such, they make mistakes in their training practices, technical application and their nutrition. Look at the diets of some well-known fighters and martial arts

action stars, and it's amazing they can perform at all, let alone do well. Here are some examples:

• Boxing champion George Foreman prides himself on eating cheeseburgers at least once a day, yet he competed against younger, stronger and faster opponents on an international level. Co-author Christensen attended Foreman's last fight in Las Vegas and says he was overweight and his punching form was terrible. Still he knocked out Michael Moorer with a punch that would have done the same to an elephant. There are a number of reasons that account for Foreman's ability to overcome his poor physicality: As a tall heavyweight, he possessed natural power in his punches and had experience boxing some of the greatest champions of his era, giving him invaluable ring experience and savvy the others didn't have.

• Consider martial arts actor Jackie Chan who we have seen perform incredible acrobatic martial arts and often bone breaking stunts. When asked in an interview about his diet, he answered, "I eat everything. Most important is training."[2] Say what? In all due respect, please don't follow Chan's poor dietary practice. We love the guy and hope he ages well in spite of his diet and on-set injuries.

• Once when co-author Demeere was coaching the Belgian wushu team at a European championship, he noticed a man in the dining hall where the teams ate. The man, in his late 30's, short and clearly overweight, always topped off his meals with several beers. Demeere assumed he was one of the coaches setting a bad example but later learned to his amazement that he was a competitor. In fact, he fought to victory in match after match, even knocking out several of his opponents. Although his last match was a tough one, he still managed to take home the gold.

• Christensen wrote an article for *Karate Illustrated* magazine several years ago about the negative impact of using marijuana (it slows thinking, reaction time and so on). A few months after the piece appeared, a top tournament competitor, a man in his late 30s, confronted Christensen and aggressively challenged the information in the article. "I smoke it all the time," he said. "I even smoked it last night at an all-night party." After the conversation, the man went on to win the tournament. Like George Foreman, he was far from the best technical fighter at the competition, but he had tremendous experience,

ring savvy and knowledge as to what it took to win at tag karate. He dropped out of sight a few years later and we hope he has retained his health.

• According to Davis Miller, author of *The Tao of Bruce Lee* and others, Lee was in terrible health the last six months of his life. Though he looked fantastic in his last picture, Enter the Dragon, his weight loss and low body fat, according to Davis, were two of many serious factors that led to his death. He squashed the assertion made by some that Lee was on a liquid diet those last months, but says he hadn't been eating well and may, according to some doctors, have had an eating disorder. [3]

The moral of these examples is that some people can do it all wrong, ignore the rules that apply to the rest of us and still be a champion. In this chapter we look into how this is possible and what it means to average martial artists.

Somotypes

A scientist (imagine Jerry Lewis in the Nutty Professor) was probably sitting on a park bench checking out passersby when he came up with the term "somotypes," since the more simplistic term, "body type" must have been, well, just too simplistic for him. He discovered there are three and the one you possess is a matter of genetic predisposition. In other words, you only have your parents to blame for not giving you a naturally ripped body. No, you can't change the genes they gave you, but that doesn't mean you can't change your appearance to some degree.

Certain fighters early in their careers possess incredibly ripped and lean physiques, but as time passes, their bodies become heavier and more muscular. People like muay Thai champion Rob Kaman or boxing champion Michael Moorer are two such examples. They began their careers lean and mean, but evolved later to heavy and mean. Their new look wasn't from fat gain but quality muscular weight, a result of changes in their training and diet. More on this in a moment.

Here are the three somotypes:

Ectomorph

Ectomorphs generally have low body fat, small bones and very little muscle mass. They are often thought of as slender or wiry and have high metabolisms that burn calories at an accelerated rate. Many ectomorphs gravitate towards endurance sports, such as long-distance running.

Endomorph

Endomorphs have large bones, high body fat and not a lot of muscle mass. If that isn't bad enough, they are cursed with a slow metabolism. It's not always easy for endomorphs wanting to participate in sports, but with effort and knowledge of nutrition and training, they can do it.

Mesomorph

Mesomorphs are the lucky guys. They have low to medium body fat levels and lots of muscle mass. Their bone size is medium to large and they enjoy a medium metabolism rate. Mesomorphs are generally natural athletes and do very well in power-oriented sports.

Before you look in the mirror to determine your somotypes, know that these are just easy labels and that it's rare for someone to fit as snug as a glove into one specific category; most people overlap. For example, your authors are endomorphs leaning toward mesomorph. You, however, might be a mesomorph leaning toward endomorph. It's beyond the scope of this book to go deeply into somotypes, and we don't have to since you need only a basic idea of the three to help you understand your body type. If you lucked out and were born a mesomorph, you should feel fortunate, but if you were born an endomorph or ectomorph, you just have to face reality and understand that you have to train harder than those lucky mesomorphs to improve your physique and turn it into a fighting machine.

Somotypes of champions

Let's say there is a champion standing before us who is a mesomorph, leaning a little towards ectomorph. He has low body fat, well-developed musculature and a high metabolism (we so hate this guy). While there are many top athletes who achieve these features through hard training, our man started out this way. He even had a six-pack and defined triceps when he was a baby. Okay, that is an exaggeration, but the point is that he has never had to put effort into his physique.

When this mesomorph began training in the martial arts, an endeavor for which he had a natural talent (are you starting to hate him, too?), he quickly developed fighting endurance, technical skill, more muscle and flexibility. Since he already had a fast metabolism that burned calories at an accelerated rate, the addition of martial arts training to his life stoked this fire even more. It's as if this guy is bathed in a celestial light and can do no wrong. It's also how he can get away with eating an absurdly unhealthy diet.

All his daily cheeseburgers, fries, beer, pop and cookies are thrown seemingly into a white-hot blazing furnace, never to show their ugly selves on his body. On top of this, his superior genetic makeup allows him to train, compete and perform superlatively despite his lousy diet.

So what happens when martial artists read an article that quotes a national champion as saying that he drinks lots of beer and eats lots of pizza just like that champ described above? What happens when fans of a martial art movie hero hears that their idol uses cocaine? The sad answer is that some will emulate their hero.

One big-name, irresponsible tournament champion, who conducts numerous seminars, brags about how he loves fast-food burgers. This from a fighter who holds advanced college degrees. It's our unasked for opinion that there is an ethical responsibility that goes along with the role of champion or movie martial arts hero. These people fought for that position and once there, they should conduct themselves as leaders under the microscope, especially when people attend their seminars to learn from them. Many do accept the responsibility, but many others don't.

George Burns Syndrome

Whenever people talk about the importance of eating a good diet and following a healthy lifestyle, inevitably someone says, "Yeah, but my grandpa ate fried food and drank beer every day and he lived to 85." Okay, the speaker has a point, not much of one, but a point nonetheless. It's true that some people can break all the rules of healthy living their entire life and get away with it. To top it off, they live longer than the average person and appear to be in perfect health. We call this the George Burns syndrome.

Comedian, actor, writer, singer, dancer - Burns did it all. He was rarely sick, worked constantly, and every day drank two martinis and smoked 15 to 20 cigars. Whenever someone asked him in his later years what his doctor said about his heavy smoking, he would answer that his doctor wasn't saying anything because he was dead. Around the age of 80, Burns appeared on the cover of Playboy magazine surrounded by a bevy of beauties. He died two months before his 100th birthday, probably with a smile on his face.

So how is it possible for some people to blatantly violate all the rules and live long, seemingly healthy lives? Uh...we don't know. Actually, no one knows.

Medical science is advancing faster today than at any other time in history. People are now able to survive illnesses and traumatic injuries that would have been fatal only 10 years ago. Still, there is so much that is not fully understood. Medical science simply doesn't know everything about disease and the effects of certain factors on the human body. It's known what increases your risks of developing a specific condition but it's also known that not everyone is affected by these risks. This is because there are so many factors involved, such as what you eat, how it's prepared, the environment in which you live, your genetic predisposition, how you handle stress, and so on. The more exposed you are to these factors, the greater the risk of incurring problems, though as we see with George Burns and others like him, it's not an absolute.

It's similar to martial arts competition where few tournament fighters go through their career without at least one loss. This is because each new match exposes the unbeatable fighter to one more competitor who just might be the one, for any number of reasons, to defeat him. For most it eventually happens, but for a rare few, despite the ever-pending risk, they maintain a flawless scorecard their entire careers. They are the George Burns of the martial arts world.

Nothing Lasts Forever

A mesomorph martial artist who eats poorly and doesn't follow any of the healthy guidelines we discussed in this book is doing a great disservice to himself now and in the long run. He might look great on the outside, but he is slowly destroying his insides. The life of a martial arts star, no matter in what area he shines, is one of hard training and continuous vigilance to stay on top. Month after month, year after year, he pushes his body to the limits of its capabilities, and then he pushes even more. Even when blessed with all that is a mesomorph, there is only so much his body can tolerate.

If he is blessed, his body might last his entire career, or if he really is mortal, it begins to fail midway. Though it can't be scientifically proven 100 percent that his eventual health problems are a result of bad nutrition and general wellness habits, it most likely is a major factor. It just makes sense: When a genetically blessed fighter pushes his body through all the rigors of the martial arts but doesn't feed it the necessary macro and micronutrients, it's going to erode and even cannibalize itself for the nutrients it so desperately needs. If he is super blessed and his body holds up until he reaches middle age, all the injuries and dietary abuse will come back to bite him, sometimes like sharks in a feeding frenzy. So many people, especially athletes, spend the last half of their lives doctoring the abuse they did to themselves the first half of their lives.

Old George smoked his first cigar at the age of 12 and was rarely seen without one in his mouth until the day he died. Why do some people die at age 40 from lung cancer but Burns smoked for over 85 years and never got it? Who knows? Might he have had a genetic potential that shielded him from the risks of smoking? Maybe. So, should you deliberately smoke like a chimney or practice your kata on the freeway? No. Likewise, when you see a champion martial artist following a diet or lifestyle that flies against all that you know is healthy, consider that he just might be the exception to the rule. You, however, might not be. For every one person who beats the odds, there are millions who don't. Since you can't see into the future, there is no way of knowing if an unhealthy habit, even a small one, will strike you down in your prime. Live your life with intelligence and with respect for the body you have been given.

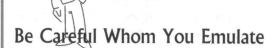

Be Careful Whom You Emulate

Two drunks are sitting in a bar located on the top floor of downtown highrise. One of them says, "You know, I can jump out the window, fall all the way down to the sidewalk and bounce all the way back up here without a scratch." The other drunk doesn't believe it so they bet each other to do it, the winner getting another drink.

The first drunk leaps out of the window, lands on the sidewalk and bounces all the way back up to the window where he lands gently on the sill. There isn't a scratch on him.

The second drunk jumps, falls all the way down to the sidewalk and lands with a *Kaaasplat!!!* Instant death.

When the first drunk orders another drink to celebrate his win, the bartender leans forward and says, "You know Superman, you can be kinda nasty when you've been drinking."

Moral: *Just because one exception to the rule can do it, doesn't mean you can.*

A Better Way

Most champions do get it though, because most aren't anomalies but hard-training fighters. They understand that there is very little difference at the top between Number One and Number Two. They know that having a bad day or having trained just a little less than their opponent can be enough to cause defeat. The skill level of fighters at the top is so high that every advantage is critical, and each one knows that if he doesn't take it, his opponents will.

The advantage of eating well is a no-brainer. While the rare champion, the anomaly we have been discussing, can get away with eating junk food and still perform outstandingly, consider this: How much harder could he train if he fueled his body with top-quality nutrients? How much better could he perform? How much faster could his injuries heal? How much longer could he compete at the highest level?

We encourage you to read about champion fighters and movie martial artists, but never emulate them 100 percent, especially those anomalies who do everything considered bad for their health. You are an individual. Read and study everything you can on health, nutrition and training, and then create a wellness and training plan that works for your particular needs. The study of the martial arts and all that it involves is about self-knowledge. Self. Yourself.

Know what works for you.

Fast Facts

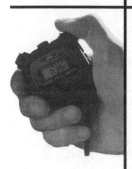

- If you have a job where you sit at a desk all afternoon or all your classes in school are lecture, your lunch should be low in calories and carbs.

- In general, complex carbs are of greater value to your martial arts because they yield more energy for a greater period.

- The "Glycemic Index (GI) is a system that rates carbs as to how fast they are broken down and sent into your bloodstream to be used as energy for your workouts.

- Always remember that your body doesn't waste much and unfortunately it doesn't discard unused calories like a dog shaking water from its coat.

- Protein and carbs both have about four calories in each gram, but all fat —saturated, polyunsaturated, or monosaturated — has nine calories in each gram.

- A rule of thumb is to consume roughly 2-3 grams of carbohydrate daily for each pound of body weight.

- Don't be fooled by "lean" or "extra lean" ground beef labels, or labels that proclaim "10 percent fat" or, "90 percent lean."

- While you should include protein in your meals throughout the day, research shows that it's vital to consume some immediately after training, specifically, within 30 minutes of your workout.

- Do 15 minutes of extra training and trim a couple hundred calories from your daily chow, and you go to bed at night with 300 to 450 fewer calories. Do this for a week and a half and there will be one less pound showing on the bathroom scale

CHAPTER THREE

All About Calories

Calories: We count them and curse them; we ignore them and try to "burn them off;" and then in our depression, we binge on them. What the heck are these little demons, anyway?

Some scientists define a single calorie as the amount of energy it takes to raise one gram of water (about a thimble full) one degrees Celsius. That is good to know the next time you want to heat up a thimble of water, but for our purposes here, let's define a calorie as one unit of energy. You need lots of units to kick, punch, grapple, spar, perform kata, and thump on the bags. You need calories to train and you need them to lie on your couch and read this text. How many you need depends on the intensity you bring to these activities: easy days require fewer units than those days when you have killer workouts. The trick is to know how many to take in.

Since we all have different bodies and we all work, study, rest, and play at different intensities, each of us has different calorie needs. If you live, train and love hard (you animal!), you need more calories. But if you are a laid back kind of person, favoring the couch over painting the garage, and tai chi over Brazilian jujitsu, you don't need as many because you don't burn as many. It's a simplification, but think of calories as gasoline you put into your car. When you accelerate hard and brake hard at stoplights, you need to refuel more often since you burn lots of gas. But when you accelerate slowly and brake gradually, you don't need to refuel as often because easy driving uses less fuel. Before we burn any additional gas or calories here, let's take a quick look at the components of nutrition.

We begin with the macronutrients: carbs, fat and protein. Knowledge of each one is important when calculating the caloric needs for your training, for your all-important recuperation and growth process after your workout and for your health needs in general.

Carbs

Carbohydrates, or carbs, are found almost exclusively in plant foods, such as fruits, vegetables, peas and beans. Milk and milk products are the only foods derived from animals that contain a significant amount of carbs. After you chew and swallow them, your body breaks them down further, converting them into blood glucose (blood sugar) to fuel your muscles, organs and brain for your daily activities, including your training sessions. An insufficient intake of carbs results in sluggish thinking and physical fatigue, attributes clearly not wanted by a hard fighting warrior.

In one study where participants were asked to exercise to exhaustion, those who ate a high-carbohydrate diet could continue exercising almost three times longer than those who ate mostly fat. [4] Even when trying to lose weight, it's vitally important that you take in enough carbs to fuel your body for all that you do in a day.

Simple and Complex

Carbs are categorized as simple or complex, which refer to their molecular structure and how the body uses them. Simple carbs have either one sugar molecule, called monosaccharides, or two molecules, called disaccharides, while complex carbs have three or more. Simple carbohydrates are usually low in nutritional quality, while complex carbohydrates are more nutritious, containing dietary fiber, vitamins, and minerals. In general,

complex carbs are of greater value to your martial arts because they yield more energy for a greater period. Here is a list of the most common in each category:

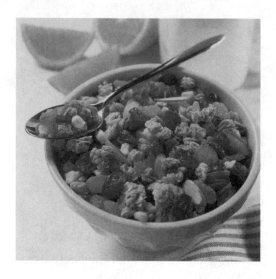

Complex Carbs

- Cereals
- Bananas
- Pears
- Whole-grain breads
- Legumes
- Nuts
- Potatoes

Simple Carbs

- Candy bars
- Cookies
- Honey
- Syrup
- White breads
- Cakes, pastry

There is nothing in the "Simple Carbs" list that you want in the finely-tuned fighting machine that is your body. We aren't saying that you need to eat like a monk and never enjoy pancakes or a chocolate bar (don't even get co-author Demeere started about the superiority of Belgian chocolate). We just encourage you to tread softly around these goodies. Maybe consider them a treat to enjoy on your Dirt Day (see Chapter 7) or, if you can justify the calories, on those days when you don't train. But they should be avoided before training and on competition day for reasons explained in the next section.

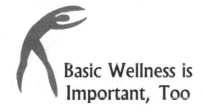

Basic Wellness is Important, Too

In your study of health and nutrition, never skip over anything that relates to your basic wellness, your basic health. We mention this because so many students don't care about their general health but are more interested in what it takes to get energy to train, recuperate, kick faster, punch harder, get stronger, and so on. They don't consider that if they aren't healthy they can't put their all into their training. Always strive for optimum health first, before you go for the extras. Your mother was right: Eat your vegetables!

Glycemic Index

The Glycemic Index (GI) is a system that rates carbs as to how fast they are broken down and sent into your bloodstream to be used as energy for your workouts. The higher a specific carb scores on this chart the faster it enters your system. Think of the listed foods in the table as a comparison against pure glucose, which is 100 percent. If a food is absorbed faster than glucose, it scores over 100 percent. While having a quick backfist is a good thing, eating carbs that quickly enter your bloodstream isn't.

After your body burns high scorers, your energy drops fast, commonly referred to as an "energy crash." This is one of many reasons why you shouldn't eat candy bars, doughnuts or other simple sugars before training or competing. They might give you a fast boost of energy, but too soon you are running on empty, with an hour left of class or an entire afternoon at a tournament. Low-scoring carbs, however, yield energy to your punches and kicks over a prolonged period, keeping your blood glucose steadier and preventing those sudden, bone weary crashes.

In his excellent book *The Science of Martial Arts Training*, Charles I. Staley, MSS writes: "High GI foods cause the pancreas to release insulin in response to the influx of blood glucose. Insulin acts to store ingested calories as body fat. This is why the GI of some foods can be surprising. For example, ice cream has a relatively low GI, because of the fat content. This means that should you get low- or non-fat ice cream, it may have a higher GI [because of the sugar added to hide the lack of flavor lost when the fat was removed, which may also supply more calories than you want] and is probably a poorer choice than the higher fat version for weight-loss purposes (although, total calorie content must also be considered.)" [5]

Carbohydrates are rarely eaten alone; most often, you eat them in combination with other nutrients, which is good. When fat, protein and fiber are eaten with carbs, the carb's GI rating drops, so that you benefit from a slower release of energy. A carb food with a moderately high GI rating, such as white spaghetti, gets a lower score when eaten with a sauce containing some fat and protein.

Note: A food's GI rating is just an analytical tool to help you choose quality foods that provide energy that lasts throughout your school or workday and into the evening for your martial arts class. Think of the GI as a pretty darn good rule of thumb rather than as a strict guideline.

Glycemic Index table

Carbohydrates that are absorbed rapidly by the digestive system

Puffed Rice	133
Rice Cakes	133
Maltose	110
Breakfast Cereal	100+
100%	
Glucose	100
White Bread	100
Whole Wheat Bread	100
90% to 100%	
Grape Nuts	98
Potato (russet)	98
Parsnips	97
Carrots	92
80% to 90%	
Rolled oats (quick)	80 - 90
Oat bran	80 - 90
Instant mashed potatoes	80
Honey	87
White rice	82
Brown rice	82
Banana	82
Potato (white)	81
Corn	82
70% to 79%	
All-Bran	74
Kidney Beans	71

Carbohydrates that are absorbed at a moderate pace by the digestive system

60% to 69%	
Raisins	64
Mars Bars	68
Spaghetti (white)	60
Spaghetti (whole wheat)	60
Pinto Beans	60
Garbanzo Beans	61
Beets	64
50% to 59%	
Peas (frozen)	51
Sucrose	59
Potato Chips	51
Yams	51
40% to 49%	
Orange	40
Navy Beans	40
Peas (dried)	49
Grapes	45
Whole Grain Rye Bread	42
Sponge Cake	46
Oat Meal (longer cooking)	49
Sweet Potato	48
Orange Juice	46
Pears	43

Carbohydrates that are absorbed slowly by the digestive system

30% to 39%	
Apple	39
Black-eyed peas	33
Chickpeas	36
Ice Cream	36
Milk (skim)	32
Milk (whole)	34
Yogurt	36
Non-Fat Yogurt	32
Non-Fat Peach Yogurt	32
Non-Fat Apple Yogurt	39
Fish Sticks (due to breading)	38
Tomato Soup	38
20% to 29%	
Lentils	29
Fructose	20
Plums	25
Peaches	29
Grapefruit	26
Cherries	23
10% to 19%	
Soybeans (high fat content retards absorption of carbohydrates)	15
Peanuts (high fat content retards absorption of carbohydrates)	13

Fruit juices

High
Banana
Moderate
Pear
Orange
Apple
Grape
Low
Peaches
Plums
Cherries
Grapefruit

Note: Since the glycemic index of each of these fruits can differ drastically, categories denoting high, moderate and low are used instead of percentages.

Ignore Carb's Bad Reputation

Unfortunately, carbs have become associated with obesity, an underserved reputation based on their easy availability. Well, ignore the rep. Carbs don't make you fat; taking in too many carbs does, because that means you are getting more calories than you need, which is the real villain that gives you a jelly belly. Follow what the old, white-bearded sage always says (the ancient master who sits naked at the entrance of high-mountain cave and says profound things all day): "Everything in moderation."

The key is to consume only the carbs you need based on your activity level. Always remember that your body doesn't waste much and unfortunately it doesn't discard unused calories like a dog shaking water from its coat. If you need 2,000 calories a day to do all your activities but you over indulge in carbs to the tune of 2,500, your body stores the extra 500 as fat. It doesn't care if the calories came from carbs or that lint that collects under your bed.

How Many Carbs Per Day?

Once again we have to speak in generalities. Though this is still a point of debate among experts, many recommend that 40 percent of your daily calories consist of carbs. Competitive bicyclists pedaling 300 miles a week require a diet of 60 percent carbs to satisfy their tremendous outpouring of energy. For the average martial artist, it's been our experience that 40 percent is a good starting point.

Now, if your job is an extremely physical one, such as a construction worker, bricklayer or high-rise window washer, and you also train hard in the martial arts every evening, you may want to nudge your carb percentage up to 45, 50, 55, or 60 percent. The same is true if you are a student dashing from class to class, including a tough physical education class, then off to an after-school job stacking crates in a warehouse, and then to martial arts training four evenings a week.

If you find yourself exhausted at the end of the day and still feeling tired after a night of sleep, 40 percent carbs might be insufficient, so you need to adjust. Do it slowly, though, adding, say, five percent every week so you can monitor the changes in your energy, progress, strength, motivation and weight loss or gain. More on this in "Protein, carbs and fat: How much?" later in this chapter

A rule of thumb is to consume roughly 2-4 grams of carbohydrate daily for each pound of body weight. If you weigh 150-pounds, you should consume between 300 and 450 grams. Pick up a book that lists carb grams (some super markets sell them in booklet form on racks by the checkout stand). If you make a habit of referring to the list every time you eat something, you will quickly memorize the gram count of those foods you eat the most often. Remember, eat mostly low scoring complex carbs on the GI chart so your energy holds constant throughout your activities.

Protein

Protein is necessary to build and repair your muscles after a hard workout and to continuously feed your tissues, hair, red blood cells, fingernails, organs and other precious parts. Once you ingest that tuna, beef, milk or nutrition bar, the protein is broken down into amino acids, of which there are 20, eight referred to as essential since your body can't manufacture them. If you lack any of the essential amino acids (a common problem with vegetarians who don't properly combine their foods to get a complete protein), your body's repairing processes suffers.

How Much to Consume

We know that you need a steady supply of protein to function at your best in your daily activities and in your martial arts training, but *steady supply* are two vague terms that for years have caused misunderstanding and debate among nutritionists, bodybuilders and martial artists. How often is steady? How much is supply?

Much of the confusion is based on a truth that says protein is vital for building and repairing muscle. Armed with just that tidbit of information, many athletes, mostly those in the more-is-better camp, think, "Hmmm. I'll eat pounds of the stuff and get really big and strong (and their super secret thought: 'and I'll be admired by both sexes and have more friends and get invited to more parties')."

3 Case Studies

Co-author Christensen used to lift weights with an NBA player and two hardcore bodybuilders. The basketball player, all six feet 11 inches of him, was a vegetarian who had been plagued with injuries for several years that would sideline him from the game days at a time, sometimes weeks. One day, the gym owner and the player sat down and discussed the player's diet, which the gym owner quickly determined was drastically low in protein. The basketball player had been making the common mistake of not properly combining his vegetables and beans, and therefore not getting all eight essential amino acids. The gym owner formulated a better vegetarian diet for him, one consisting of complete protein and an overall greater volume of it. The next year, the NBA man played injury free for the first time in years, and his team went on to play and win the NBA championships, in which he was the high scoring star.

One of the two bodybuilders worked as a police officer, 220 pounds of traffic-stopping muscle as he walked his beat with every bulge rippling through his uniform. To pack on a few more pounds of muscle in preparation for the Mr. America contest, he increased his already-high protein intake to two and a half grams for each pound of his bodyweight, an amount suggested by the makers of the protein supplement. Within months, he was hospitalized with critical kidney damage. The cause, the doctor said, was his body's inability

to handle the excessive volume of protein.

The other bodybuilder was 190 pounds of hard, ripped muscle. Not believing the one or two grams of protein per pound of bodyweight theory, he decided to see how low he could go and still progress. Over the course of 18 months, he slowly and progressively dropped his intake to 30 grams a day (about one gram per six pounds of bodyweight) - all the while continuing to pack on muscle.

The how much dilemma So how do you know what to believe? For sure there is a lot of confusing information out there. Go to a local health food store and the clerk says you should drink a protein shake with each meal. Read the label on the protein powder canister and it instructs you to mix two scoops in water or milk and drink three servings a day (hmm, think that just might be a ploy to get you to use up a can of the stuff every three days). The "experts" at the gym advise you to drink protein shakes and chow down on as much chicken, cottage cheese, beef and milk as your bloating stomach can handle. The folks with diplomas on their walls, the sports medicine people, dietitians, and such, tell you to eat only a moderate amount of protein. It's enough to make you go to a diner and order a big piece of pie with two scoops of ice cream.

You might be getting enough right now. Most athletes, with the exception of some vegetarians, are already eating enough protein without having to sit down and do the math. Every day, they consciously or unconsciously eat a little extra chicken, tuna and drink a glass or two of skim milk. In fact, most people consume protein-heavy diets, which is true even for those who haunt the greasy burger joints on a regular basis (no, we are not recommending greasy burger joints).

4 Ways to Calculate Your Needs

As a thinking martial artist who recognizes that good eating habits account for much of your progress, you need an easy way to calculate your protein intake. Well, you came to the right place; in fact, here are four easy ways to determine your daily requirement.

Method one: This method is based on a general guideline that puts your daily protein need between .03 and .09grams of per pound of bodyweight. Here is how it looks for a 150-pound fighter and a 200-pound fighter.

150-pound fighter

.03 x 150 = 45 grams of protein per day

.09 x 150 = 135 grams of protein

200-pound fighter

.03 x 200 = 60 grams of protein

.09 x 200 = 180 grams of protein

Yes, .03 to .09 is a large margin, but every person is different so you have to experiment to see what works best for you.

Method two: With this, you multiply your bodyweight times .36 grams to determine your daily intake. This is the formula used to calculate the Recommended Daily Allowance (RDA) found on food labels. For most martial artists who train regularly, this supplies an adequate daily intake; but it should be considered the absolute minimum. Let's use our 150- and 200-pound friends again.

150-pound fighter

.36 x 150 pounds = 55 grams of protein

200 pound fighter

.36 x 200 = 72 grams of protein

Method three: This method for determining your daily protein need is called the "Hatfield Estimate," a unique formula that takes into account your lean body mass (LBW) and your activity level, referred to as your Need Factor (NF).

LBW: Your lean body weight is your weight minus your body fat. Since fat doesn't require protein, there is no need to calculate your total body weight. To get an estimate of your LBW, you need first to determine the percentage of body fat you carry around. This is done using ultrasound or electrical impedance, methods used by many commercial gyms and by sports medicine doctors and dietitians.[6] Call one of these places and ask to have your body fat measured and calculated in pounds. You can also purchase skin fold calipers, though they are less accurate. That said, Christensen once had the task of using skin fold calipers to measure the body fat of over 1000 police officers. His calculations were within one to two percent of those officers who had had their body fat measured by more high-tech means. That is good enough for our purposes.

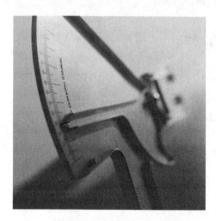

Once the short procedure is completed, subtract the fat poundage from your total body weight and the answer — *tu-duh* — is your LBW. Here is an example using a 150-pound person with 30 percent body fat.

.30 X 150 = 45 pounds of body fat.

150 - 45 = 105 pounds of lean body mass

Need Factor: The NF is your best guesstimate of your activity level; use the below scale to give it a number. Be honest about your activity level so you know exactly how much protein to take in every day. Should you rate yourself too high you will end up taking in more protein and calories than you need.

.5 - Sedentary, no sports or training

.6 - Jogging or light fitness training

.7 - Sports participation or moderate martial arts training three times a week

.8 - Moderate weight training, aerobic or martial arts training daily

.9 - Heavy weight training daily

1.0 - Heavy weight training daily and martial arts training daily

Take your NF number and multiply your LBW to determine your daily protein requirement in grams. The math looks like this: LBW x N F = daily grams. If you are as bad at math as we are, toss your calculator out the window and use this chart that does it for you.

Weight	Need factor and corresponding protein requirements					
LBW (lbs)*	.5	.6	.7	.8	.9	1.0
90	45	54	63	72	81	90
100	50	60	70	80	90	100
110	55	66	77	88	99	110
120	60	72	84	96	108	120
130	65	78	91	104	117	130
140	70	84	98	112	126	140
150	75	90	105	120	135	150
160	80	96	112	128	144	160
170	85	102	119	136	153	170
180	90	108	126	144	162	180
190	95	114	133	152	171	190
200	100	120	140	160	180	200
210	105	126	147	168	189	210
220	110	132	154	176	198	220
230	115	138	161	184	207	230
240	120	144	168	192	216	240

Examples If your LBW is 90 and you have determined that you have a need factor of .9, you need to consume around 80 grams of proten a day. If your LBW is 240 and your NF is .5, you need to get 120 grams of proten a day.

Method four: Since this approach requires that you experiment to find what works and what doesn't, you must be in tune with your body as to how it feels before, during and after your training sessions. It's helpful to maintain a log to note other data, such as how you feel the day following a hard workout, or whether you lost, maintained, or gained energy, strength, and endurance. Your log should include the amount of protein you consume daily and how you felt upon making changes, say when you added 20 grams or eliminated 20 grams.

Note As you experiment carefully as to the best dosage for your body relative to the demands on it, it's important to keep in mind that all four of these methods are only close estimations of your daily protein needs. Also, the benefits of using a log are not restricted to Method Four. Many fighters find it helpful to keep records of their intake so that they have a visual record to help them compare how they feel before, during and after training.

When Should You Eat Protein?

While you should include protein in your meals throughout the day, research shows that it's vital to consume some immediately after training, specifically, within 30 minutes of your workout. Your second best option is to eat it within the hour, and your last choice is to eat it within two hours after you train. We encourage you to arrange your schedule so you can get protein in your system within 30 minutes, since your body so desperately needs it to repair all the "tearing" down you did. It's never an option not to eat protein after your training. When you don't refuel your body properly, the repairing phase might be incomplete or delayed, both of which puts you at risk of overtraining or getting injured when you use muscles in your next workout that have not yet recuperated.

Your Post Workout Needs

There are nutritionists who recommend you eat carbohydrates — such as a banana, apple, or a slice of nutrition-rich bread — after training to replenish your energy stores. We agree with this, but with an explanation. Yes, you do need to jump start your energy with carbs, but you also need protein to repair tissue damage done in your training. If your workout was mostly aerobic, such as high-repetition drills and lots of wind-sucking sparring, you should eat mostly carbs and just a little protein afterwards. If your workout consisted of weight training only, or your sadistic instructor made you do sets and reps of horse stance squats and lots of pushups, you need more protein and less carbs. Whatever the combination, the blend of carbs and protein compliment each other for faster absorption, which is why most protein shakes contain a small amount of carbs.

The best post-workout protein are those that are easily digested, such as eggs, lean fish, lean chicken, and whey protein shakes. Steak, on the other hand, while high in protein (and lots of bad fat) is hard to digest, especially when your body is already working overtime to recuperate from your workout.

Everyday Foods High in Protein

Here are some typical protein foods you want to include in your daily diet.

- Meat, poultry and fish — 7 grams per ounce

- Beans, dried peas, lentils — 7 grams per 1/2 cup cooked

- One large egg — 7 grams

- Milk — 8 grams per cup

- Bread — 4 grams per slice

- Cereal — 4 grams per 1/2 cup

- Vegetables — 2 grams per 1/2 cup

Protein Supplements

Many nutritionists argue that there is no real advantage to taking protein supplements, advice which few hard-training athletes adhere to. Dr. Susan M. Kleiner, R.D., Ph.D., a nutritionist and the co-author of *Power Eating*, says, "There's no advantage to taking protein as a supplement. It's not absorbed better. It's not utilized better."[7] In fact, as co-author Christensen's bodybuilding friend discovered the hard way, extra protein may over time put stress on your kidneys (one sure sign you are eating too much protein is when your kidney blows out your lower back and rolls down the street like a dislodged hubcap).

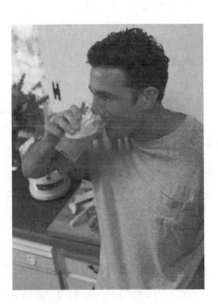

How we do it   Here is how we use protein supplements: Demeere, who is on the run all the time visiting clients, likes protein milkshake replacement meals combined with a little fruit. He drinks them in the car while en route to a client, or at the end of a hard day when he needs some extra repair fuel. Christensen always has a scoop in a glass of water after a workout. On those days when he doesn't eat meat, he sprinkles a tablespoon on his cereal or in his yogurt to get an extra 15 to 20 grams. We especially like that many protein supplements are fortified with vitamins and minerals, a nice plus when using them as a meal replacement or to punch up a container of yogurt.

Regardless of what the gym rat advises (the guy with veins in his forehead who goes "Huh?" a lot), if your calculations show you are getting enough protein from your food, you don't need to take a supplement. However, it's still a good idea to keep a container of supplemental protein in your cupboard for those days when your hectic lifestyle prevents you from getting the grams you need.

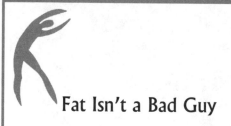

Fat Isn't a Bad Guy

Besides its use as an energy source, you need fat to maintain healthy skin, carry fat-soluble vitamins (A, D, E, and K) into your body, support your immune system, insulate you against the cold, cushion your internal organs, and make food taste better, which all adds up to mean that fat is not the bad guy some experts want you to believe.

Fat

Although fat has a bad reputation, it's actually a secondary fuel source. When your body runs out of carbohydrates to use as energy, it draws energy from fat, which yields about nine calories per gram, compared to four calories per gram of protein and carbs. The average person has enough carb energy in his body to walk about 20 miles, but he has enough fat energy to walk from Boston to San Francisco three times (go ahead and do it; we'll be here when you get back).

While your body likes to store fat as an extra "fuel tank," far too many people, including too many martial artists, carry around fuel tanks that are much too large. This would be acceptable if you were running about on the plains tackling and killing bison for the village all day, but that is not the kind of life you lead (except perhaps for our Wyoming readers).

In an effort to keep things simple, let's classify fat as either saturated or unsaturated.

Saturated Fat

Saturated fat is generally solid at room temperature and found in animal sources, such as dairy products, meats, fish, lard, butter, hard margarine, cheese, whole milk and anything in which these ingredients are used, such as cakes, chocolate, biscuits, pies and pastries. It's also the white fat you can see on red meat and that stuff lurking underneath poultry skin. Consume an excessive amount of saturated fat, and you get an increase in "bad" cholesterol (LDL), which can lead to heart disease and cancer.

Unsaturated Fat

The so-called "good fat," is usually liquid at room temperature and generally comes from vegetable sources. Monounsaturated and polyunsaturated fat are both included in this group. Unsaturated fat is a healthier alternative to saturated fat and can be found in vegetable oils, such as sesame, sunflower, soya and olive oil. It's also found in oily fish, such as mackerel, sardines, pilchards and salmon. Peanut butter contains the good oil, too, as do most nuts. When choosing a peanut butter, get the kind that contains only ground nuts, and avoid the kind that includes several unpronounceable chemicals. Although all of these foods contain the good fat your body needs to stay in optimum health, you still need to eat them in moderation since they are so very calorie dense: nine per gram.

Free tip 1: Plan to gorge on a high-fat meal tonight? Think about this first. Studies show that several hours after you eat a meal containing 50 to 80 grams of fat, your blood vessels become less elastic and there is a dramatic rise in factors that lead to blood clotting. "The immediate cause of most heart attacks is the last fatty meal," says William Castelli, M.D., director of the Farmington Cardiovascular Institute in Massachusetts. [8] It's much healthier for you to spread your fat intake over the entire day.

Psst, for males only: Studies show that a high-fat meal isn't good for your love life either as it may lower your testosterone level. We aren't going to get in to that here, but just know that if you want to be a fighter and a lover, a big fatty meal could be your downfall.

Always keep in mind, and yes we harp on this a lot, your body stores all excess calories as fat, whether they come from protein, carbs or fat. If the calories don't get used, they make you feel like a cow when performing your kata.

On that note, let's talk about how to slice a pie, a big chocolate cream pie with tons of whipping cream and chocolate shavings on top. Yeah, right. You wish.

Slicing the Calorie Pie

You just learned why protein, carbs and fat are essential to your training and progress. Here is a simple pie chart that helps you split your nutritional needs as your training dictates.

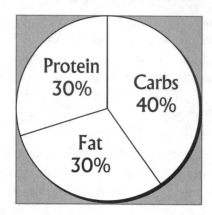

Many athletes base their daily nutritional plan around portions that are 40 percent carbs, 30 percent protein and 30 percent fat. This means that if a fighter were following an eating plan of 2000 calories a day, his slices would look like this:

40 percent carbs:	800 calories
30 percent protein:	600 calories
30 percent fat:	600 calories
Total:	2000 calories

But as is the case with everything in the diet and training field, the sizes of these slices has been a debate in nutritional circles for a long time and probably will remain so in the future. Over the years, your authors have tried many different sizes, which have led us to this conclusion as to how large each one should be: It depends. (This won't be the last time we give a wish-washy answer.)

Several years ago, co-author Demeere had what he describes as a painful pie-slicing experience. After he quit competing internationally and had reduced his training to about one third of his competitive schedule, he made the common error of continuing to eat as if he still trained four to six hours a day, burning 3,000 to 3,500 calories. He also ate foods that had been forbidden in his hard training diet: sugar-dense chocolate, soft drinks and many meals of fat-laden steak smothered in cream sauce with a truckload of french fries. In short, his fat and carb slices were much larger than his protein slices.

Two things occurred to him one day: Over a five-year period, his poor eating had added around 30 pounds, and in a few months there would be photos taken at his wedding. Not wanting a memory album picturing a chubby groom, he knew he had to drop the bulk that he had had so much fun accumulating.

He went to a highly recommended doctor who promptly put him on a low-carb diet consisting of 1,500 calories a day and supplied him with herbal supplements, assuring him that they would give him energy for his two-hour-a-day workouts. Skeptical, he asked numerous questions, which she patiently answered with quotes from so-called "scientific studies."

Since the balance of carbs, protein, fat and calories were so poorly prescribed (the carb slice was virtually nonexistent) his once easy daily training regimen of 30 minutes aerobics and 30 to 40 minutes of weight training, in addition to six-days-a-week, two-hour martial arts sessions, became grueling. He burned 1500 calories quickly in his training, which left him without energy for the rest of his day. He felt weak, saw black spots dancing in front of his eyes, and his carb-depleted brain throbbed with a continuous and horrendous headache.

Clearly, you shouldn't experience these symptoms when dieting. If you do, consider it nature's way of telling you that your diet advice was lousy, if not dangerous. Yes, Demeere lost the extra pounds he had been packing around (and the pictures turned out great), but he was only successful because he stopped following the doctor's ill-advised diet after four weeks, and used one of his own.

Everyone Has an Opinion

If you research five nutritional sources you will find five different ways to slice the pie, but don't let that frustrate you. Understand that none of this is set in stone, meaning that what works for the star black belt in your school or the guy on the magazine cover, might not work for you. So what will? Well, to avoid being the sixth nutritional source, we are simply going to give you the

information you need to figure it out for yourself.

First, determine your calorie needs and then slice your pie 40 percent carbs, 30 percent protein and 30 percent fat. Stay with it for a month to see how you feel. Take note of your energy level, how quickly you recover from your training, your mental sharpness, how motivated you are for your next training session, and whether you are progressing in power, speed and endurance. If you are dragging in all these areas, you need to change your slices a little.

Here are a few considerations to help you establish the right cuts:

- Don't listen to what others are doing. Think only about your needs. As we discussed earlier, emulating others is a common error in the fitness world. Don't do it.

- Think of carbs as your main source of energy, but remember, adding protein and fat to your meals lowers the glycemic value of the meal and provides for longer lasting energy. Try to include all three macronutrients whenever you eat.

- The percentages change depending on all the factors in your training. Sometimes you might have special carb needs. For example, if you attend a weeklong, martial arts seminar where you train eight hours a day, you might want to increase your carbs for your extra energy needs. Refer to the chart that lists calories per hour per martial art to determine a ballpark number as to how many extra calories you need for the long training days.

Say, you determine that you need an extra 1000 calories. This means you must increase your carbohydrate cut of the pie from 40 percent to 60 or maybe even 70 percent. Of course, when the carb slice increases in size, the protein and fat slice has to get smaller. So if you increase to 60 percent carbs, divide the protein and fat evenly at 20 percent each. It's a good idea to increase your carbs to 60 or 70 percent at least once before the date of the training camp so you know in advance if your body can even assimilate that many carbs without problems. Making emergency runs to the restroom on your first day isn't a good way to make an impression.

- If you want to hit the weights extra hard for three months to put on additional muscle size and increase your strength, you need larger slices of protein. To determine how much more, monitor your gain in lean muscle weight by measuring your fat percentage (as discussed earlier) to get an idea of your progress throughout the three months. Then use the previously mentioned Hatfield chart to calculate how much protein you need on a daily basis (see Chapter 11 for more details on increasing muscle size). When taking a larger protein slice, rob the extra calories from the fat piece.

- Know that your body doesn't like radical changes and it will protest. Say you have been taking in 60 percent carbs because you have been training for a running marathon in addition to your regular martial arts workouts. The marathon is over, and now you want to decrease your carbs back to your starting point of 40 percent or wherever you were before increasing your training. Do this slowly, changing a little each week. From your starting place of 60 percent carbs, drop to 55 percent the first week, 50 percent the next week, 45 the next, and to 40 percent the week after that. Avoid bigger increments.

- Make your nutritional plan for tomorrow, tonight. Here are some considerations:

  ☐ If tomorrow is a day off from training, plan to eat fewer carbs and calories.

  ☐ If tomorrow is your regular martial arts class and your regular daily activities, use the calculations you figured earlier.

  ☐ If you have a regular day tomorrow at school or work, but you have a three-hour test for brown belt tomorrow night, plan on taking a little larger slice of carbs.

  It's easier to stay on your plan when you work this out a day in advance.

- Allow for unforeseen situations. Since life has a tendency to interfere with your schedule — you can't eat at the times you want, or the grocery store is out of your favorite protein — plan for such obstacles in advance.

- People who make the greatest progress almost always keep a meticulous training log. At first, you might think that it's time consuming and not much fun, but after a couple of weeks, you will probably discover as others have that it's invaluable for staying on course. It provides you with all the necessary tools to determine your maintenance needs and provides a clear picture of which direction you need to change, if at all. Use the sample logs in the back of this book or use the format to develop one of your own.

- Check regularly to see if your ratios still hold true today as they did two months ago. You might have gained some extra muscle mass over an eight-week period, so you need to factor in a little more protein, say 40 percent of the pie. Maybe you have been pushing yourself harder during sparring sessions and therefore you need more carbs, say a 50-percent slice. Count on your dietary needs changing occasionally.

Vitamins and Minerals

Vitamins and minerals create healthy blood cells, maintain healthy skin, regulate your metabolism, ensure that your brain works, strengthen your teeth and bones, and many other valuable functions. Since they don't make up an important part of your caloric intake, we won't elaborate on them here but we will go into greater detail in Chapter 5 as to how much you need of each and their importance for martial artists. For now, know that they are critical for staying healthy as you work to lose, maintain or purposefully gain weight.

Determining the Calories Needed to Gain, Lose or Maintain

Here is a simple and effective method for calculating your daily caloric needs, one recommended by health and fitness writer, Dave Paicard, which he discusses in an article titled "Basic Strategies for Getting Lean" in *Muscle & Fitness Online*.[9] It's not absolutely precise (no system is) but considering all the variables, it's pretty darn close and serves our purpose. We have tweaked it a little to make it applicable to martial artists. Check out these bullets and see where you are:

- To lose fat, multiply your current bodyweight by 10 if you have a slow metabolism (meaning you gain weight easily), by 11 if you have a moderate metabolism and by 12 if you have a fast metabolism (meaning you can eat lots without putting on weight).

- If you incorporate weight training in your exercise program and you want to add muscle without body fat, or if you lift weights and want to lose some body fat, you need to multiply your body weight by 13 if you have a slow metabolism, by 14 if you have a moderate metabolism, or 15 if you have a fast one.

- If you are trying to add a few pounds, multiply your weight by 16 if you have a slow metabolism, by 17 for a moderate metabolism, or 18 for a fast metabolism.

Confused? Here it is at quick glance:

Fat loss formula: bodyweight (pounds) x M (metabolism) = total daily calories

Metabolism rate: 10 for slow, 11 for moderate, 12 for fast

Muscle gain without fat formula: bodyweight x M = total daily calories

Metabolism rate: 13 for slow, 14 for moderate, 15 for fast

Weight gain: bodyweight x M = total daily calories

Metabolism rate: 16 for slow, 17 for moderate, 18 for fast

Here is how it looks for a 130-pound female with a moderate metabolism. She is pumping iron to add muscle for greater kicking power and wants to lower her body fat at the same time.

130 x 14 = 1,820 calories per day

Here is how it looks for a 200-pound male with a fast metabolism wanting to add muscle without fat to increase his punching power.

200 x 15 = 3,000 calories per day

Note: To make this work accurately, you need to be honest about whether you have a slow, moderate, or fast metabolism. If you are like some people, you might think you have a slow metabolism because you think you gain weight easily, but you actually eat a lot of hidden calories that you aren't taking into account. You do this by:

- adding a little extra butter on your toast

- eating that last cookie so it doesn't go to waste

- drinking milk instead of water when you are thirsty

- eating what is left in the skillet instead of putting it into a refrigerator container

- eating just a little bowl of ice cream

- drinking a second beer

In time, these not so innocent extras add up, and while you might not be aware you are eating them, they are definitely there, encircling your waistline and adding droop to your "buttline." In the end (pun intended) you don't have a slow metabolism at all.

We suggest that you do two things. First, get an opinion from your doctor as to what type of metabolism you have. Second, keep an accurate record of everything — everything — you eat in a week. That t-spoon of jam you snuck: write it down. You finished your kid's fries: write it down. You ate a cookie you found on the street: write it down.

If your record keeping and your doctor indicate that you do indeed have a slow metabolism, then you need to calculate your calorie needs as such. However, if you determine that you have been taking in a lot of extra sneaky ones, you need to calculate using the moderate formula. You have to be honest here. It's like Mrs. Beasley said in third grade: "If you cheat, you only cheat yourself."

One Other Way Men and Women Are Different

Do men and women burn calories differently? Many women believe so, especially when they look at men who are the same age and body type as they are but the men seem to shed unwanted pounds faster and easier. Many female martial artists complain that it seems that all they have to do to put on

unwanted weight is to slack off on their training a little, but the same doesn't hold true for most men.

What is going on? The answer is simple: Men and women have different bodies. (Now, aren't you glad you bought this book?)

The biggest difference, for our purposes here, has to do with muscles. In general, men have more muscle mass than women, and the person with more muscle mass burns more calories. Even when sitting still. This is because it takes calories to maintain the muscle.

When a man and woman of the same body type, age, weight and activity level eat too much at a fast food joint, the man usually stores less excess calories as fat than does the woman. And his larger muscle mass will burn off his excess calories faster.

Women think this is unfair and men think it's just fine. But there is a silver lining for women. Generally speaking, their higher body fat percentage is considered, in most cultures, to be more attractive on them than the same percentage is on most men.[10]

Calculating Your Caloric Needs for Training

Use the following list to calculate the calories needed per hour for your particular martial arts style, and if you jog and lift weights, you can calculate those in, too. Don't engrave the data presented in this chart on a stone tablet. It's difficult at best to determine calorie expenditure because there are so many variables (no, those gauges on treadmills aren't absolutely accurate, either). The numbers in the below chart have been calculated with a formula for the average male and female fighter, not for a top martial athlete or a rank beginner.

This chart, and others like it, has been calculated using bodyweight and duration of activity as the primary, determining factors. However, there are many more factors that are beyond the scope of a simple chart: intensity (an elite kickboxer usually trains harder than a novice), the fighter's lean muscle tissue, bodyfat percentage, height, age, sex, food consumed that day, quality of the previous night's sleep, and many others. Adding factors makes for an extremely complex chart, one that is not only difficult to read but one that is more complicated than most fighters need for reference. While ours is a compromise between accuracy and simplicity, the absence of more

Calories Burnt Per Hour Per Activity
Martial Arts Chart

Activity	110-pound	125-pound	150-pound	175-pound	200-pound
Boxing: sparring	493	552	610	669	727
Boxing: bag work	330	368	407	446	485
Kickboxing	548	613	678	743	808
Karate	467	532	620	742	850
Taekwondo	430	520	610	715	800
Tai Chi	201	233	262	297	323
Judo	509	579	678	743	808
Jujitsu	509	579	678	743	808
Weightlifting	306	348	407	504	576
Running: 6 m.p.h.	509	579	678	840	960

variables makes it a tad less precise. Still, it provides you with a general idea, a so-called ballpark figure that serves as a starting point for you.

Should you notice that you aren't losing body fat or you are having trouble gaining lean muscle, re-calculate how many calories you need and increase or decrease the numbers on this chart, but only a little. For example, the first time increase or decrease only 100 calories, and if that doesn't help in two or three weeks, increase or decrease 200.

Use the training logs at the back of the book. They provide a great visual to see where you need to make adjustments in your training intensity and your calorie intake (most often it shows that you simply have to train a little harder and take in a few less calories).

The information on this chart has worked for martial artists for many years. However, if you think the data is too general for you because you have a need to know exactly how many calories you burn, go to a professional sports testing facility or see if your local university has the proper equipment. At those places, you will find equipment and trained professionals who can give you accurate data. However, be prepared to spend a chunk of money as these tests tend to be expensive.

1 2 3 A Simple Primer to Losing Weight

You are going to get lots of easy-to-follow eating plans later to lose weight without hunger. Here is one you can start right now.

Eat a little less   Simply cut back 200 or 300 calories each day. For example, if you normally eat three slices of bread per day, cut back to one slice and don't put butter on it. Drink diet soda, or better yet drink water. You don't want or need to eliminate massive amounts of calories and you certainly don't have to go hungry. By cutting calories sensibly and conservatively, you barely notice you are eating less than normal.

Train a little more   Next, do 15 extra minutes of training — kickboxing, running, kata practice, bag thumping — to burn another 100 to 150 calories.

That is all you have to do: 15 minutes of extra training and trim a couple hundred calories from your daily chow, and you go to bed at night with 300 to 450 fewer calories. Do this for a week and a half and there will be one less pound showing on the bathroom scale. Oh yes, the extra 15 minutes of training makes you just that much better in your fighting art. It's a pretty good deal.

More on this in subsequent chapters.

Fast Facts

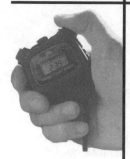

- Carbohydrates are the fuel that feeds your engine and keeps you training when your instructor calls for 50 more reps.

- There are many carbohydrate diets that either limit how many grams you eat or make them more important than other vital nutrients. Neither extreme is good for a hard training martial artist.

- Numerous low carb/high protein diets are currently in vogue. Do keep in mind that while some might have merit for losing weight, they aren't targeted at athletes, but rather at obese and sedentary individuals.

- Be aware that some low-fat packaged foods contain extra sugar calories for flavor. Don't assume that "reduced fat," means reduced calories.

- Your body stores fat as a secondary source of energy. Once you burn up your carbs, your body draws on stored fat to get you through your day and training.

- High-protein diets deprive your brain of glucose, which it needs for normal functioning, such as thinking and maintaining fast reaction time.

- For a martial artist, the worst reaction to sudden, harsh calorie restriction is the loss of lean muscle.

- The essential component in most fad diets, no matter what bizarre scheme they take, is the reduction of calories.

- When liquid diets are used to replace two or more meals, you might not get sufficient nutrients, which isn't an option since as a martial athlete you need all you can get.

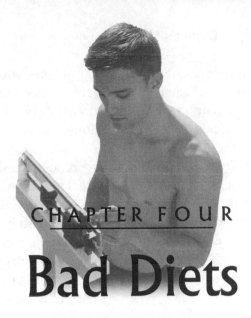

CHAPTER FOUR

Bad Diets

Why Low-carb, Low-fat & Low-protein Diets are Bad for Martial Artists

Over the years, there have been many low-carbohydrate or low-fat diets promoted as the answer to the woes of people long struggling to drop a few pounds. For the most part, these have been fad diets that, in some cases, have been dangerous even for people who don't exercise, and terribly dangerous for people who make great demands on their bodies in the martial arts. To understand why, we need to look closely at the functions of these macronutrients.

Carbohydrates

As mentioned in Chapter 2, carbs are the primary source of energy for your body. They are the fuel that feeds your engine and keeps you training when your instructor calls for 50 more reps. When you ingest carbs your body converts them into blood sugar (glucose) to be used in every endeavor requiring energy, everything from combing your hair to punishing a heavy bag. If your body doesn't use all the energy, it converts and stores it as glycogen in your muscle cells and liver; think of it as an energy reserve. Problems arise when you eat carbs to refill the depleted glycogen stores in your muscles after training, but you eat more than you need so that there are calories left over in the form of glucose. Since your muscles and liver are full, the only place for that extra glucose to go is into fat. When that happens, the seams of your training uniform begin to cry for mercy and dogs bark as you pass by.

Keeping your muscles full of energy requires that you constantly replenish them with carbs. It takes about 24 hours after a hard workout for your muscles to refill completely with glycogen, provided that you take in a sufficient amount to do the job. If you don't take in enough, and you train again the next day, you begin with a glycogen supply that is already low. Should you do it again on the third day, again on the fourth and so on, you will soon suffer from chronic fatigue. This happens routinely to people on extreme diets.

Low-carb Diets

Training in the martial arts is a combination of physical and mental skills, all of which require sufficient energy to function at their optimum. The source of this energy comes from carbs, the same ones that some anti-carb diets restrict.

It's important to eat a meal of carbs before your training session so you have enough glucose and glycogen stores to get you through the rigors of kicking and punching. If your workout is a tough one and you didn't eat enough carbs to support your energy needs for the entire session, you might feel like one of co-author Christensen's students who had been following a low-carb diet. Half way through a particularly hard class he groaned picturesquely, "I feel like warmed over puke."

Since your brain needs the energy it gets from carbs to think clearly, to remember things such as the moves in your kata, and to perceive the world as a happy place, an excessively low-carb diet punishes you with irritability, a throbbing headache and an inability to concentrate and focus, not only in your training but at work and in school.

If you choose to shed body fat via your martial arts training, you have to experiment to find a happy balance with your carb intake. Know that there is going to be a tradeoff: You don't want to eat more carbs than you need because that makes you chubby, and you don't want to eat too few carbs because you won't have sufficient energy to train hard enough to burn off your love handles. You have to experiment to see what is right for you, but don't fret over it. Read on because we give you some ways to make the struggle doable.

Carbohydrate Diets Are All About Calories

There are many carbohydrate diets that either limit how many grams you eat or make them more important than other vital nutrients. Neither extreme is good for a hard training martial artist.

Too few and your training suffers
Since carbs are an important source of what keeps you going, eating a diet that severely restricts them poses a major problem when you want to train long and hard or do well at an all-day tournament. Without sufficient carbs, you can't perform at your best, you tire quickly and, in time, you might become ill. Your carb-starved body might even break down your own muscle fiber to

use as energy, meaning that you literally cannibalize yourself. Then one morning when doing your regular biceps flexing in the bathroom mirror, you scream in horror at what appears to be limp spaghetti hanging from your shoulders. That is a bit of an exaggeration, but not much. Read on.

Several years ago, co-author Christensen competed in the Mr. Oregon bodybuilding championships (yes, he wore those skimpy little posing trunks and smeared his body with oil, but that's another story). Being naïve and misinformed, he followed a Spartan diet consisting of tuna fish, turkey and one orange a day. As the orange was his only source of carbs, his energy took a nosedive, as did his strength. After three months, his bodyweight was down 30 pounds, his muscles had shrunk and his strength had depleted to the extent that he could barely manage 35-pound dumbbells for bench pressing; 90 days earlier he had been using 115-pounders. Not only did the dramatic reduction in carbs make him feel miserable for those three months, in the end he lost the contest.

When you deplete your glycogen stores following a low-carb diet, your body turns to other sources for energy, namely fat and protein. While it's desirable to burn fat as fuel, protein should be spared. We have heard many students say that they don't care if they lose some muscle because they just want to be thinner. We disagree, and here is why.

When you run out of a glycogen, your ravenous body cannibalizes your muscles of amino acids and sends them to your liver. Once there, they convert into glucose and move into your bloodstream to fuel your working muscles. This isn't good since the theft of your amino acids attacks the very thing you use in your training: muscles. By using protein for energy, you remove what your body needs for growth and repair of muscle tissue, thus slowing and endangering your recuperation, and ultimately hampering your progress.

To put it into training terms: You can say goodbye to the crispness of your forms, your power on the heavy bag, your speed when sparring, and your motivation to train. There is nothing you want by restricting your carb intake to the extent that your body eats itself. Think of it this way: Carbs are nutrients that "spare" protein.

When you lower your caloric intake of carbs in the extreme, you have to increase your intake of fat or protein. If you need 2000 calories a day and cut out 500 calories of carbs, you still need those 2000. So you have to replace them with more fat or more protein. Increasing your fat intake isn't a good option, and increasing your protein intake too much can be hazardous to your health. Too much protein has been associated with liver and kidney problems, loss of bone density, dehydration and arthritis.

Low carbs are not for athletes
Numerous low carb/high protein diets

are in vogue as we write this. Do keep in mind that while some may have merit for losing weight, they aren't targeted at athletes, but rather at obese and sedentary individuals. As a martial artist, your dietary needs are different from those of a couch potato's. You need more energy, more protein and more water for the rigors that you put your body through.

Too many and you get chubby A different problem arises when you consume an excessively high amount of carbs, say, 70 to 80 percent of your daily calorie intake for several weeks in a row. We have said repeatedly that when you take in more than you need for your energy expenditure, your body stores the excess as fat. If that isn't bad enough, there is research that paints an even bleaker picture. Ron Kennedy M.D., author of *The Thinking Person's Guide to Perfect Health*, writes: "Excess carbohydrates also causes generalized vascular disease. The high-carbohydrate diet, which is now so popular, causes the pancreas to produce large amounts of insulin, and if this happens for many years in a genetically predisposed person, the insulin receptors throughout the body become resistant to insulin. Because insulin's action is to drive glucose into the cells, this results in chronic hyperglycemia, also called high blood sugar. A large portion of this sugar is stored as fat resulting in obesity. Excess insulin also causes hypertension and helps initiate the sequence of events in the arterial wall, which leads to arteriosclerosis and heart disease." [11]

Let Your Activity Determine Your Intake

If you have a job where you sit at a desk all afternoon or all your classes in school are lecture, your lunch should be low in calories and low in carbs. If you have a job that is physically demanding or you have a rigorous gym class in the afternoon at school, your lunch needs to contain enough calories and carbs to supply your body with sufficient energy. If you know your evening martial arts class is going to be a hard, two-hour session, make sure you eat enough quality carbs in the afternoon to last you until the final bow. If you study tai chi, or you know your taekwondo or karate training is going to be an easy session, then eat a meal of moderate calories and carbs.

To lose, maintain, or gain weight, you need to be cognizant of your body's fuel needs for your specific lifestyle. A lifestyle with moderate activity gets a moderate number of carbs, while an active lifestyle gets a greater number. Say you have an intense martial arts class on Monday, Wednesday and Friday, but Tuesdays and Thursdays you sit at a desk all day. On Monday, Wednesday and Fridays, therefore, you should eat more carbs to satisfy your greater energy needs, and fewer on Tuesday and Thursday.

We can't give you the exact number of carbs because there are so many variables involved with each individual. Your best bet is to study the charts we have provided to determine your caloric and carb needs for your activity level. While this might seem like a big hassle at first, it's worth the effort to do the simple math, and after a week or so, you will have developed an intuition as to what works for you.

Does Anyone Carbo-load Anymore?

The concept of carbo-loading has been around for some time and remains a controversial subject in training circles and in the medical community. Endurance athletes, like runners, competitive swimmers, and bicycle racers use it to provide long lasting energy. Some bodybuilders engage in carbo-loading as a way to make their bulked muscles look more defined for a short while, such as for posing competition or a photo shoot. But is it for martial artists? We don't think so.

How it works To carbo-load, you deliberately take in and store more glycogen than you do normally. One method is to first suffer through a depletion phase for at least two days, eating only fats and proteins and little or no carbs. It's advised that you continue to train during the depletion phase, though you feel rundown, a little like fresh road kill. Training hard helps to speed up the carb depletion phase by burning all of your body's reserves. After two to seven days of this, you happily gorge on all the carbs you want - spaghetti, brown rice, apples, potatoes, and good breads. Since your body has been carb depleted, it's starved for glycogen, and it stores more than usual before turning the excess to fat.

Carbo-loading bodybuilders find that glycogen is absorbed directly into their muscles, giving them a fuller and more voluminous look. Now this may be fine for looking buff for a couple of days, but it doesn't do anything for your martial arts practice. Actually, it's a terribly unhealthy state for bodybuilders and it's not uncommon for a competitor, as a result of extreme dieting, overtraining and purposefully dehydrating himself, to collapse during the show.

"Wow, that bodybuilder just passed out up there on the stage."

"Yeah, but he sure looks good."

Again, there is nothing in that that you want. Besides, martial arts aren't about looking good but about learning physical and mental skills. That said, when your nutrition is up to par, by following the advice in this book, a happy byproduct of your training is that you will likely develop a muscular, lean body.

For marathon athletes, carbo-loading after the depletion phase is supposed to fuel the body's glycogen stores to their maximum, reducing the runners' need to eat during the race. Re-fueling in the middle of an event can be hard on one's digestion, which can ultimately affect performance.

Training during the depletion phase Here is another reason we aren't in favor of carbo-loading for the martial artist. To obtain the best results in the glycogen uptake, you need to deplete your current glycogen stores, which is usually accomplished through exhaustive training sessions. During this phase, you can't punch and kick at your usual best and, most likely, you are going to be tired, drained and wiped out. There is no way around this because it's part of the carbo-loading process, but it's one that is dangerous. When glycogen is depleted, you are one tired fighter and ripe for a training injury, especially if you are preparing hard for a lengthy belt promotion exam or a big all-day tournament. It's understood that in martial arts circles it's common to "push the envelope" to see how far one can go to strengthen that can-do-never-quit mindset, but do you really want to blow a shoulder two days before the big day because of poor nutrition? Do you really want to blow a shoulder anytime?

Case study Demeere used to study a hard Chinese style called Hung chia pai, an art that draws heavily on physical strength and incredible endurance. After several years of training, he was asked to test for his teacher's degree. The main portion of the test took over six hours to complete, and a seventh hour required him to sit in a low horse stance for a full 60 minutes. Just before he had to endure the horse stance, he was told to spar three rounds using Sanda rules, a mix of kickboxing and stand-up grappling. The only sustenance he had during these long, torturous hours were a few slices of bread during a brief lunch break and water every 15 to 20 minutes. Bread and water isn't a diet conducive to optimum physical performance and clear, rationally thinking.

He faired well during the first round, but then he executed what he refers to as "the stupidest move I have ever done in my life:" He blocked a roundhouse kick with his face. Too tired and drained to think clearly and judge the attack accurately, he leaned toward the kick, instead of moving his head away, and collided painfully with his opponent's hard shinbone. Fortunately, the kick was not as fast or as powerful as it could have been, but it still broke his nose, requiring surgery. To this day he has an ongoing hearing problem from that missed block.

Your brain needs glucose to function optimally. If it doesn't get the stuff, it begins to malfunction, doing funny things like moving into an attack. There is no place for fuzzy or slow thinking in the martial arts as the nature of the game is to make split second decisions: dodge the blow or block it; attack or backpedal; throw a combination or a single technique; and so on.

Demeere looks back on his test and believes that a major factor of his fatigue was a result of his poor nutritional strategy. He didn't eat properly during the test and he should have been drinking sports drinks instead of plain water. He learned his lesson the hard way and isn't about to repeat that error, since a broken nose and corrective surgery really hurt.

If you still need convincing not to carbo-load, consider what exercise physiologist and nutrition consultant L. Lee Coyne, Ph.D. says: "Elevated carbohydrate intake increases the insulin production which increases fat storage, interferes with fat mobilization for energy, disturbs other hormonal balances, and increases blood pressure, blood cholesterol and triglyceride levels. Carbo-loading can aggravate hypoglycemic responses during team sports and this can impair judgment, concentration and other performance measures." [12]

There is no reason for you to carbo-load. Most martial arts training sessions are stop and go events and most competitions consist of several bursts of all-out effort with rest periods in between. It's far more advantageous to follow a sound daily nutritional plan as presented in this book and then eat intelligently for your event.

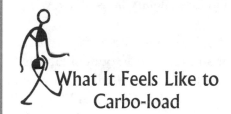

What It Feels Like to Carbo-load

People with low tolerance for consuming large quantities of carbohydrates during a single meal, complain of nausea, stomach bloat, lightheadedness and fatigue. Carbo-loading runners often say on race day that they feel heavy, a by-product of extra water stored in the muscles with the extra glycogen, so much that it could increase one's bodyweight two to three percent and cause muscles to feel stiff.

Feeling terrible the last few days before an event and on the big day, won't help to get you into the right mindset, especially when you are already struggling to contend with stress, which is busily sapping your precious energy. Some athletes experience stress a week before the event, some a day before and some a few hours before. Add a carb depletion phase to all this and you have a whole other category of discomfort to contend with, symptoms often described as similar to a cold or flu.

Bottom line: You won't be a fun person to be around on the big day, especially when it affects your performance.

Fat

To our minds, fat is a bad thing. The mighty leap to this conclusion goes something like this: When I eat too much dietary fat, I gain too much body fat. Therefore, dietary fat is bad.

Well, there is some truth to this. When you eat an excessive amount of fat-filled foods but fail to burn off all the calories, cruel people make "Goodyear Blimp" comments behind your back. But don't conclude from this that all dietary fat is bad and that you should therefore eliminate it from your diet. In this case, one truth doesn't equal another. The real truth is that your body needs it, and without it, you would soon become ill, so ill that you could possible die. Strong claim? Yes, but nonetheless a truth. Here is why:

• As noted earlier, fat is critical to the absorption of certain vitamins, such as A, D, E and K, which are called fat-soluble because they need fat to do their jobs in your body.

• Fat provides you with essential fatty acids (EFA), nutrients your body desperately needs but can't manufacture by itself. Fail to get enough EFAs and you get low energy, dry skin, hair loss, kidney, liver and brain degeneration, attention deficit disorder, depression, poor wound healing, sterility, miscarriage, arthritis-like conditions, heartbeat abnormalities that can lead to cardiac arrest, and growth retardation in children. In other words, you aren't a happy camper.

• Your body stores fat as a secondary source of energy. Once you burn up your carbs, your sweaty body draws on stored fat to get you through your day and your training.

Still want to eliminate all fat from your meals? We hope not, because you need it to achieve all that you want in the martial arts. The tricky part, however, is that if you consume too much, you counteract your training efforts. Making it even trickier is that it's so darn easy to consume too much. Grrr, why can't things ever be easy?

Remember, there are nine calories in a gram of fat, while protein and carbs contain only four. Think of that the next time you shovel down a whipcreamed-covered chocolate pie or a big ol' sauce-loaded, drippy hamburger (double grrr: Why is all the good stuff bad for you?). Unless you draw on that martial arts discipline, you can easily go into "fat overdrive."

Even low-fat foods can be a problem if you aren't careful. You may indeed be eating less fat, but remember that low-fat doesn't mean low calorie since many of them are filled with sugar to overcome the icky taste of the missing fat (triple grrr). So don't look only at the "low-fat" data on the label, check out the calories, too.

More on the Two Fats

As we discussed in the last chapter, all fat is not created equal. There is saturated fat, found mostly in animal sources, such as meat, milk and butter, and there is unsaturated fat, found in vegetable sources, such as olive oil, peanuts, corn and other nuts and seeds. Saturated fat has been linked to illnesses, especially cholesterol problems, like arteriosclerosis or "plaque buildup" in the arteries. This means that arteries get clogged and your heart has to work overtime to do its job correctly.

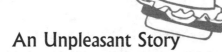

An Unpleasant Story

Co-author Christensen once talked with a nurse whose job was to assist doctors in conducting autopsies. She said over her many years on the job, she had seen more and more teenagers with severe artery plaque from what she believed to be their ever increasing intake of fast foods. She said it was common now to find deceased teenagers (who had died from accidents, illnesses, or homicide) with so much hard plaque in their arteries that she has to use a hacksaw (a saw used to cut metal) to cut through them. More and more, the arteries of fat-guzzling teens are becoming similar to those of people in their 70s and 80s. Think of that the next time you order a super-large container of double-grease dipped fries with your greasy burger.

Think unsaturated Strive to eat mostly unsaturated fat since it can actually help to prevent all the bad done by saturated fat. Unsaturated fat has even been known to lower the risk of certain cancers. So right now, go toss out that saturated butter and replace it with unsaturated olive oil. Use olive oil for cooking and as a salad dressing instead of that toxic vegetable oil. If you eat out often, you will happily find that because more and more people carefully monitor their cholesterol, many restaurants now note in their menus that certain foods have been cooked with olive oil.

There are even good "butters" on the market now (most are called "spreads" that contain olive oil) and note on their labels that the product helps fight heart disease. Choose one that contains more monosaturated fat than saturated and polysaturated fat. For example, we have a spread right here in front of us that contains one gram of saturated fat, two grams of polyunsaturated and four and a half grams of monosaturated fat. Four and a half grams is the highest mono we have found. There are no sugars or cholesterol in ours, and it's really quite tasty. In fact, with many of these healthy spreads, it's impossible to differentiate them from real butter. You know, if we all switched to butter-like spreads that contain high monosaturated fat, we would soon put all the cows out to pasture. (Sorry, couldn't resist.)

Be careful, because even the good fat is high in calories. If you start packing extra spread on your corn-on-the-cob, you will soon pack extra spread on your butt. Remember what the old sage says: "Everything in moderation."

Fat Diets Are All About Calories

Since one gram of fat contains nine calories compared to four calories in one carb gram and one protein gram, simple math tells us it's twice as easy to take in too many calories when following a high-fat diet. Ingesting excessive fat will only add fat to your body, not to mention placing you at risk of various cardiovascular diseases. In other words, you look bad and feel like crud.

Fat diets have been all the rage lately, but results have been mixed. An underlying assumption with many of these diets is that carbohydrates are bad, so to avoid these naughty macronutrients, the dieter eats mostly protein and fat. We don't want to get technical as to what happens inside your body when following this plan because we don't like it and we don't want to give it much space here. In a nutshell, the idea is to make fat a primary ingredient in your meals so your body uses it as its energy source.

This might sound like a good concept, but it has a few inherent problems. One concerns the negative impact that a high-fat diet has on your cholesterol level. High cholesterol, often called the "silent killer," is one of the major causes

of death throughout the world. Remember, you want more unsaturated fat and less saturated. When you increase fat in your diet at the expense of eating carbs, it's difficult to ensure that your fat intake is mainly from unsaturated sources. Fail, and you place your health at risk.

Another issue is that of food selection. High-protein, high-fat diets steer you away from vegetables and fruit that supply fiber, vitamins and minerals. Some companies that encourage these diets advise that you take supplements to counter this. Now, here is a surprise: many of these companies just happen to sell the exact supplements you need.

The micronutrients found in fruits and veggies play an important role in keeping your body running in top form. As a martial athlete, you need even more of them since your intense training rapidly depletes your reserves. If you don't replace them and then train again the next day, and again you don't replace them and train the next day...how long do you think you can keep this up before something on your body breaks, or worse, falls off? Okay, nothing is going to fall off, but you get the idea.

No-fat Diets

Some diets go in the other direction and eliminate all fat. A no-fat diet would be counterproductive in the long run since, as discussed earlier, you need it to assimilate fat-soluble vitamins. You might get away with cutting fat for a while, but eventually you are going to suffer. For your body to function at its best, you need about 30 percent of your daily caloric intake to be fat. You need to focus on eating mostly unsaturated fats and as always you need to count your calories. Make it your lifestyle to drink skim milk; choose baked and broiled foods over fried; remove all visible fat from beef, turkey and chicken; use fruit spreads instead of butter and learn to enjoy low-fat cheeses. Cut the bad fat, eat the good fat, but don't go over 30 percent.

When You Have to Reduce Your Fat Slice

On those occasions when you want to increase the size of your carb slice from the pie because you have a rigorous training schedule, or increase your protein slice because you are hitting the weights extra hard for a while, reduce your fat intake to 20 percent, even 10 percent, but never longer than a few weeks.

The Bad News About Protein Diets

There are high-fat and low-fat diets, high-carb and low-carb diets, so it stands to reason that there are high-protein diets, which usually follow the same line of thinking as high-fat diets: carbs are bad. The literature is inconsistent as to what constitutes a high-protein diet, but most experts say that you are at risk if it consists of over 40 percent of your daily calories. Here are some of the problems you risk when going overboard with protein:

- Osteoporosis and other types of bone deterioration

- Calcium deposits

- Dental decay

- Stomach and digestive troubles

- Stiff joints

- Gout

- Circulatory and blood pressure troubles

- Kidney and bladder stones

Most who follow a high-protein diet are also taking in a tremendous volume of fat (the exception are those folks getting their protein from vegetable sources). Three ounces of hamburger, for example, which is quite small by most people's standards, contains about 22 grams of protein, 20 grams of saturated animal fat and oodles of gooey cholesterol. Many followers experience an elevation in their LDL (the bad) cholesterol when they remain on the diet for long periods. High levels of LDL cholesterol and clogged arteries are the chief culprit of heart disease, heart attack and stroke. One slight "advantage" to a high-protein diet is that the large amount of fat you get with it helps you feel full faster so you just might eat fewer calories. Might. But it's not worth it health-wise.

Calcium Loss and Brittle Bones

High-protein diets place big-time stress on your kidneys since they have to work overtime to assimilate the stuff. Should you follow such a diet for several months, you just might experience a toxic goodie in your body called urea, which is a by-product of protein metabolism. To get it out of your system, your body has to force more water through your kidneys to "hose them out," if you will. A negative side effect of hosing is a pronounced loss of minerals, including calcium, a critical nutrient that a body-slamming martial artist needs. The body loses an average of 1.75 milligrams of calcium in the urine for every one-gram increase in animal protein ingested. A reduction of this all-important mineral (because of poor diets millions of people already are deficient) and you risk osteoporosis, also known as, "brittle bones." This is especially prevalent in women and is nothing you want as a martial artist since you spend a lot of time whacking your bones on a mat and against training partners.

Affects the Brain

High-protein diets deprive your brain of glucose, which it needs for normal functioning, such as thinking and maintaining fast reaction time. Do we really need to say that having a good reaction time is important to you? You know you have been on a high-protein diet too long when your training partner punches, retracts his fist, adjusts his belts, sniffs, and cracks his neck, all before you go for the block.

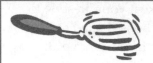

Christensen's Experience

High-protein diets aren't new. There was a popular one in the early 1970s that co-author Christensen tried for about a month. The diet was meat only, no fruit and no vegetables, not even a stick of gum. They made a point of the gum to show how critical it was to maintain the diet's protein-only regimen. Christensen stuck to it religiously for three weeks but then his "faith" started to waiver. First was the absolute drudgery of eating only meat. "Oh good. Tuna for breakfast again." Then there was the overall body weakness, making it difficult to get through even an easy workout. Then there was the problem - remember, there is no fiber at all in this diet - that prevented him from having sunshiny mornings, if you understand what that means (hint: he was constipated for nine days. Nine!). After four weeks, he switched to another diet.

All Fad Diets Are about Calories

The aforementioned carb, fat and protein diets all fall in the category of so-called fad diets. Usually they become popular after someone writes a book on the wonders of eating pork all day or drinking seaweed cocktails with every meal. A few years ago there was one that claimed beer and steak was the way to go and another that advocated wine and cheese. Lots of people happily followed these, not really caring if they lost weight.

Usually what happens is that the author gets a few disciples (remember, any diet works as long as there is a restriction of calories), makes an appearance on Oprah, and soon after everyone is following the newest craze (read: crazy). Often, the diet plan has little scientific foundation, though it's carefully designed to make its creator obscenely rich (we're so jealous). Remove all the ludicrous claims and phony testimonials and you won't discover anything special about it because it's based on the simple principle that fewer calories equate to a smaller belt size. It usually goes away about as fast as it arrived, leaving in its wake many disillusioned and still porky people.

Full-contact fighting champion Frank Shamrock says, "You have to keep away from the fad diets, the so-called latest discovery in diet technology that's going to turn you into a lean machine overnight... The trick is to eat cleaner.

We know what's good for us and what isn't. It may be fashionable to start your day with the latest state-of-the-art meal supplement, but what's wrong with a chicken breast and some white rice, or a bowl of oatmeal and a couple of eggs?" [13]

It's worth repeating, the essential component in most fad diets, no matter what bizarre scheme they take, is the reduction of calories. Whether it's three squares a day of whale fat, or the cottage cheese and grapefruit diet, they all work as long as you eat fewer calories per day than you burn in your activities. Even if you could tolerate eating such ridiculous regimens, your hard-training body would suffer since a limited variety of food equates to a lack of balanced nutrition.

Types of Fad Diets

Most fad diets fall into one of the following categories:

- **Extremely low calorie-diets**
  These are often called "crash" diets because they abruptly and extremely restrict calories, sometimes as few as 800 per day. Since some hard-training martial artists need over 3,000 calories a day, such a diet quickly depletes your energy and desire, leaving you nutritionally deficient and prone to injury. Extremely low calorie diets should be used only for a short duration and only under medical supervision. Never attempt to follow one on your own.

- **Questionable diets**
  These are diet plans that call for you to eat one specific nutrient, food, or combinations of foods. While these restricted calorie diets may lead to weight loss, they teach poor eating habits, cause nutrient deficiencies and are difficult for even the most disciplined to follow for long. By eating many different foods, you maximize your intake of all the necessary macro and micronutrients.

- **Flexible diets**
  By limiting fat intake, caloric intake or both, you choose what to eat and how much. These diets often fall short by not taking into account the totality of your body's needs. For example, some programs limit fat intake but don't consider the number of calories in the allowable carbs and protein. Eat too many calories from them, even though you reduced your fat intake, and Mr. Evil blubber stays on.

- **Formula diets**
  These are generally liquid diets such as protein shakes, various juice concoctions, and so-called meal-in-a-can diets that replace one or more of your regular meals. If used to replace two or more meals, you might not get sufficient nutrients, which isn't an option since as a martial athlete you need all you can get. Formula diets work as long as there is a reduction of calories (we have known people to drink diet shakes with a big piece of chocolate cake), but they are only a short-term solution, as people tend to regain the weight once they stop using them.

In subsequent chapters, we talk about how good eating habits are a major factor in keeping your weight normalized. Fad diets don't teach good habits because they offer only quick solutions. You might lose a few pounds, but once you have reached your desired weight and stop following the diet, they all come screaming back, and sometimes they bring extra fat friends with them. With the abundance of fad diets on the market, there are many people today suffering from health problems associated with the "yo-yo effect," a problem discussed in a moment. First, here are some dead giveaways to help you spot a fad diet.

How to Spot a Fad Diet

- If the claims are too good to be true, they probably are. Don't buy into the marketing scam that allows you to "eat all you want while you lose fat effortlessly." Few people are able to do this (we hate them). The rest of us have to work hard at it — for as long as we live. Keep in mind that there are no magic bullets or miraculous shortcuts that lead to lasting results.

- Most pills, potions, liquid diets, fat burners, and so on aren't effective or are only a short-term solution. More times than not, they waste your hard-earned cash and strain your body.

- Movie stars aren't dietitians, so why would you follow their advice? Besides, many just lend their name to a diet that has been developed by someone else. We know of one big-named actress/model who once said she could eat anything and never had to exercise. Still, she came out with an exercise and diet video when such videos were the big craze.

- Beware of claims that a diet is "scientifically proven." Oh yeah? What studies proved it? What are the names of the scientists? At what institutes? If there was a study, who or what company funded it? Be especially suspicious of studies ordered by or funded by a company to validate its own product. Was the study even conducted on people? Some products are sold with their outrageous claims backed by scientific studies, but the studies were conducted on lab rats. (Sure, the rats have attractive little bodies now and awesome sidekicks, but that doesn't mean the same diet will work for you.)

- Discard useless information. Know that a diet isn't more effective because it (1) was created by an obscure tribe in the Amazon jungle; (2) it has only recently been discovered in some exotic location; (3) it's a breakthrough in the medical field; (4) it used to be expensive but now it's available to common mortals. These claims and others like them are irrelevant and are only clever ploys by marketing people working hard to separate you from your cash.

- If an advertised diet offers a guaranteed weight loss and claims that you won't regain it, avoid it like a teen-ager avoids a lawnmower. The only guaranteed weight loss method is to spend 21 days on a raft at sea without food. A guarantee makes the product appear absolutely wonderful, and marketing people know that most consumers don't return ineffective products, anyway.

- Exercise is crucial in achieving and maintaining a happy number on your bathroom scale. Those diets that claim it's not necessary to work out are appealing to lazy consumers by telling them what they want to hear. You should wonder what other misinformation they are imparting.

Yo-yo Effect: Dangerous Weight Fluctuations

The so-called yo-yo effect is a common manifestation of crash diets, those poorly designed eating plans that call for you to drastically reduce your caloric intake. At this writing, there is a popular diet making the rounds that has people drinking a juice concoction for three days. No food, just disgusting tasting juice sold in a fruit jar. In the end, the juice drinkers are supposed to lose up to 10 pounds. While that sounds wonderful, 10 pounds are far too many to lose in such a short period. There are many reports of people suffering from nausea, weakness and dysentery from the harsh regimen (running desperately to the toilet is one way to lose weight, but do you really want to?) and making matters worse, their lost weight returns in a quick hurry when they resume their normal eating habits.

In Chapter One, we listed several other stress reactions your body has to a sudden and drastic reduction of calories. One that is terribly ironic occurs when your body goes into famine mode and sends a desperate message to your metabolism to hold on to every precious calorie it does get. This often results in no weight loss at all and sometimes a weight gain.

Goodbye Precious Muscle

For a martial artist, the worst reaction to sudden, harsh calorie restriction is the loss of lean muscle. Not only do you want every fiber of muscle you can get to slam home powerful punches and kicks, lean muscle mass is also a major player in burning more calories. Since muscle tissue has high-energy requirements, the more muscle mass you have, the more calories you burn, even when sprawled on your sofa surfing channels.   According to the American Council on Exercise, every pound of muscle burns about 50 calories a day. When you lose muscle mass from improper dieting, you have to lower your daily calories even more because you no longer have the same muscle mass to feed. More calorie cuts mean even more muscle shrinkage. It's at this point when many dieters consider taking that proverbial long walk off a short pier.

Let's say you dieted away 10 pounds in two weeks on a crash diet. Maybe you needed to fit into that slinky red dress...let's change that to you had to make weight for a competition. Never mind that you felt so wasted that you lost your first match, now that you have gone off the crash diet, your weight is climbing back up — and fast. If prior to your diet you needed 1800 calories a day to maintain your weight and satisfy all your energy needs, you now need only 1500 because you lost so much muscle. So, if out of habit you go back to eating those 1800 calories, or more since you are starving after the dramatic food restriction, and you haven't increased your training routine, the 300-calorie difference starts to pack on the lard. Before you can say, "Extra sour cream, please," you have gained your original weight back and more. This is the primary reason why so many fad diets fail, and do so miserably.

Dangerous to Your Health

On top of their ineffectiveness, the resultant yo-yo effect, when done repeatedly, places your health at risk. Case in point: There is great concern in the Hollywood medical community about actors and actresses losing and gaining weight rapidly for movie roles.

Your body doesn't like big changes because it's designed to maintain the status quo. So a sudden and major dietary change shocks it, causing it to struggle to adapt and keep all the internal parts running smoothly. Even if it does adapt, the sudden shock most certainly causes negative reactions, such as the aforementioned nausea, dysentery and other fun things.

We don't recommend extreme accelerated weight loss methods. Throughout this text we offer only sound and sensible methods to lose or gain weight for long-term results that are healthy and beneficial to your progress in the martial arts. We believe it's vital that the method fit your lifestyle because that is the only way to get results that last.

Fast Facts

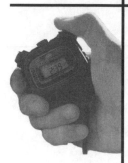

- Although the word vitamin is derived from "vitality," vitamins actually have no usable energy of their own. Without them, though, your energy wanes and you plod and stumble along like a hard-ridden horse.

- You need to eat about 1,800 calories a day to get the necessary vitamins and minerals for good health and optimal martial arts performance.

- Know that there is no scientific research that proves extra vitamins give you an edge in training or competing.

- It's best to first get your vitamins from a variety of foods before you start popping pills, as food contains other important substances that make vitamins work better.

- Since vitamins are not regulated by the federal government, there is no agreement as to what is meant by claims of "super potency," "maximum," "mega," "high potency," "stress formula," and "men's formula."

- Since so many foods today are fortified with vitamins, you might be amazed to discover how many you are already taking in.

- When it comes to quality control, the big brand names generally score better than some small manufacturers, which of course you pay for at the register.

- Since fat-soluble vitamins are stored for long periods — some stay for a few days, others for up to six months — there is a risk of toxicity should you take more than you need.

- Natural vitamins tend to be expensive since it's so pricey to extract them from natural sources. The solution? Don't buy them.

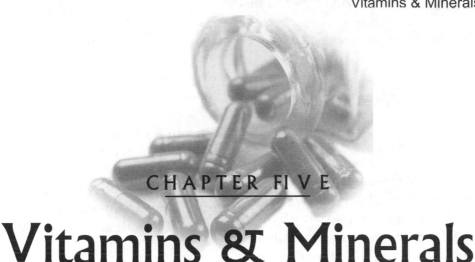

CHAPTER FIVE

Vitamins & Minerals

There have been many books written about vitamins and there is always at least one article, usually more, in each of those health and exercise magazines that crowd the newsstands. This is a good thing and we encourage you to read as much as you can on the subject so you can make informed decisions, especially since there is so much misinformation floating around and so much new data continually coming out. Our approach here is direct and simple information targeted at you, the martial artist. Nonetheless, you should consider what follows as basic information and a starting point for your particular needs.

Although the word vitamin is derived from "vitality," vitamins actually have no usable energy of their own. Without them ,though, your energy wanes and you plod and stumble along like a hard-ridden horse. This is because the existence of vitamins in your body makes possible a wide array of complex processes that create energy. Vitamins also make possible cell function, muscle

and bone growth, blood formation, and brain/muscle interaction, all of which you desperately need to punch and kick at your very best. The bottom line is that your mother was right: You need your vitamins. The tricky part is to determine how many.

Vitamin supplements are popular among athletes of every ilk: bodybuilders, runners, gymnasts, football players and martial artists. Research shows that while athletes use vitamins differently than couch potatoes, it's not clear whether this means they need more vitamins or will perform better if they increase their intake. Nonetheless, it's believed that as many as 75 percent of all athletes take some type of supplement, ranging from a simple multivitamin to a complex assortment of pills. Demeere, for example, takes one multivitamin a day, while Christensen takes a multivitamin, and additional vitamins C, E and calcium. Are we doing the right thing or are we wasting our money and only feeding the fishes some really expensive urine?

What are Vitamins?

Vitamins are an organic substance, present in minute amounts in natural foods. All 13 are essential to normal metabolism. Since your body can't manufacture vitamins, the only way it can get them is through your food and through supplements. You need to eat about 1,800 calories a day to get the necessary vitamins and minerals for good health and optimal martial arts performance. Since most fighters eat more than 1,800 calories, some nutritionists believe that vitamin and mineral supplements are needed only in special situations. For example, if you follow a vegetarian diet or you never drink milk, then you might need a supplement to make up for the vitamins and minerals you aren't getting.

Warning Should you cut back drastically on your food intake, especially below the 1,800 calorie level, you risk not getting enough vitamins and minerals, as well as an insufficient number of carbohydrates to get you through your day and your training.

Here are the 13 known vitamins along with a sentence or two as to what they do for you and in which foods you can find them.

Vitamin A (retinol) is necessary for healthy eyes, skin and the linings of your digestive and urinary tracts, and your nose. Vitamin A is found in milk, dried apricots, squash, carrots, spinach and various fortified food products.

Vitamin B1 (thiamin) helps transform carbohydrates into energy. Food sources include potatoes, fish, bananas, ham, chicken, bread, cereal, and enriched rice.

Vitamin B2 (riboflavin) is necessary for energy release and for healthy skin, mucous membranes and nervous system. Food sources include spinach, steak, cottage cheese, milk, oranges, apples, enriched bread, and enriched cereal.

Vitamin B3 (niacin) metabolizes carbohydrates, fats and proteins during the digestion process to unleash important nutrients. It's found in tuna, potatoes, halibut, peas, cereal, corn, mushrooms, peanut butter, ground beef, and enriched bread.

Vitamin B6 is necessary for the synthesis and breakdown of amino acids and helps in the metabolism of carbohydrates. You can get Vitamin B6 in peanut butter, chickpeas, chicken, spinach, cereal, potatoes, bananas, and lima beans.

Folic Acid is necessary for the production of blood cells and a healthy nervous system. Find it in spinach, broccoli, green beans, peas, lentils, asparagus, mushrooms, lima beans, and oranges.

Biotin is needed for metabolism of carbs, protein and fat. Food sources include nuts, split peas, eggs, cauliflower, and mushrooms.

Pantothenic acid is needed for metabolism of carbohydrates, protein, and fat. You find it in eggs, peanuts, mixed vegetables, steak, fish, wheat germ, and broccoli.

Vitamin B12 is needed for synthesis of red and white blood cells and the metabolism of food. It's found in chicken, meat, eggs, milk, and yogurt.

Vitamin C is necessary for healthy connective tissue, bones, teeth and cartilage. It also enhances your immune system. Food sources include bell peppers, broccoli, strawberries, oranges, potatoes, tomatoes, and kiwi.

Vitamin D is needed for calcium and phosphorus metabolism, and for healthy bones and teeth. You can get it in fortified milk, fortified cereal and sunlight.

Vitamin E is necessary for nourishing and strengthening cells. It's also an antioxidant. Food sources include sunflower oil, wheat germ, sunflower seeds, almonds, and whole wheat grain.

Vitamin K is necessary for blood clotting. Food sources include cabbage, spinach, broccoli and kale.

Water Soluble Vitamins

Vitamins C, niacin, folic acid, biotin, pantothenic acid, and the B-complex vitamins are water soluble, and as such aren't stored to a great extent in the body. This means you must take them every day. As a martial artist, it's critical that you get these nutrients, since one of their functions is to assist the work of important enzymes, including those involved in the production of energy from carbohydrates and fats.

Fat Soluble Vitamins

Vitamins A, D, E, and K are fat soluble, meaning that your body stores them in your liver and fatty tissues. They are eliminated from your body much more slowly than water-soluble vitamins. Since fat-soluble vitamins are stored for long periods — some stay for a few days, others for up to six months — there is a risk of toxicity should you take more than you need. [14]

Do Fighters Need Additional Vitamins?

Know that there is no scientific research that proves extra vitamins give you an edge in training or competing. Now, if you eat poorly — say, your daily diet consists of a loaf of toast and a meaty bone — a sudden influx of vitamins will definitely improve your training and your quality of life. Since most people eat better than this, vitamin deficiencies are usually related to various medical problems, such as anorexia, unhealthy weight loss, and malabsorption, meaning your body has trouble absorbing the good nutrients. If there were a deficiency, it would have to occur for quite some time since vitamins A, D, E and K stay in your body for a while, and even some water-soluble vitamins don't leave immediately.

We highly recommend that you take daily vitamins, but take extra large dosages of vitamins only at the direction of a doctor or sports medicine nutritionist.

Vitamin B War Story

One of Demeere's students suffered from an ongoing neck problem, a result of a bad whiplash received in a car crash. To add insult to injury, he received a hard head blow sparring, which started a tingling sensation in his left elbow. Over the next few weeks, the sensation progressed to numbness and then to a loss of his fine motor skills. Extensive medical tests showed that a major nerve had virtually wasted away due to blocked vertebrae. The student consulted numerous specialists, all of whom said he needed neck surgery. Finally, one doctor suggested an alternative, one that involved treatment with vitamin B. Three months after he had begun treatment, the nerve had fully recovered and his arm was once again functional. The doctor said the problem had been made worse by the student's vegetarian diet, which lacked sufficient B vitamins, thus leaving him susceptible to nerve damage.

Food or Supplements: Which are Better?

It's best to first get your vitamins from a variety of foods before you start popping pills, as food contains other important substances that make vitamins work better. The problem is that in today's crazy, fast-paced world, many people don't eat a balanced diet, or if they do, they don't do it all the time. Even your disciplined authors have the occasional meal of beer, a fried steak sandwich with cheese, side of fries and hold the coleslaw.

Fortified Foods

Since so many foods today are fortified with vitamins, you might be amazed to discover how many you are already taking in. For breakfast you eat a bowl of vitamin-enriched cereal along with vitamin-enriched milk and a couple of pieces of vitamin-fortified toast. You haven't even left the house and already you walk with a rattle from all the vitamins in your body. But the day is young. At midmorning, you chow down on a vitamin-enriched energy bar, and at lunch you have a sandwich made with two slices of that same vitamin-fortified bread you had at breakfast. Oh, and that cup of soup you packed? Fortified. At mid-afternoon, you have a big latte and a sugary doughnut. Okay, those things aren't fortified, but they sure are good, aren't they? At dinner you have a glass of milk fortified with vitamins, another

slice of fortified bread along with your usual meal. After your workout, you have a vitamin-fortified sports drink.

Even if a good many of the vitamins in these foods were destroyed from cooking, old age, toasting, exposure to air, sunlight, heat and cold, you are still getting a ton of vitamins. Some nutritionists say you are getting too many, while others argue that you still need to fortify in some capacity.

Super-duper, Mega Vitamins

Since vitamins are not regulated by the federal government, there is no agreement as to what is meant by claims of "super potency," "maximum," "mega," "high potency," "stress formula," and "men's formula." We encourage you to read labels and the advertising claims with a raised eyebrow of suspicion and don't automatically plunk down your change for a bottle of "super" or "mega."

For example, we saw a bottle of "women's formula" that contained the exact same number of vitamins and equivalent potency as a bottle of multivitamins two shelves down. The jar for women, however, was $10 more. Some of the so-called specialty vitamins are special only in name and higher price. Pause to read the labels and more times than not you find a so-called "stress" vitamin contains the same ingredients as the one labeled "super." By the way, there is little evidence that the stresses of daily living deplete vitamins from your body. Hmm, you would think the manufacturer would know that. Maybe they just want your dollar.

Can You Overdose?

Can too much of a good thing be harmful? Can you take too many vitamins? Yes, the problem is that it's not clear what is meant by too many. It's hard to know where to draw the line between safe and excessive micrograms, milligrams or international units because for many vitamins there isn't an officially established limit for maximum doses. We have a fairly good idea what the United States recommended daily allowance (USRDA) is at the low end, but the information is fuzzy as to what it excessive. Also, the danger levels vary from person to person, depending on the individual's body weight, health status, metabolism, diet, the vitamin in question, and how often it's taken.

We strongly urge you to follow the USRDA of vitamins, and under no circumstances take excess amounts before you consult with a nutritional expert. Some people suffer toxicity at even low dosages, while others can take greater amounts without harmful side effects. Co-author Christensen, for example, has taken what might be considered mega doses of vitamin C for years — 1,500 - 5,000 milligrams a day — without harmful side effects. Other people, however, suffer stomach problems from just 100 milligrams of vitamin C. Early on Christensen studied vitamin C at length, learning as much as possible about it, the good and the potentially bad. Today, he takes a daily dose of 1,500 milligrams, progressively increasing to 5,000 at the onset of a cold (which he rarely gets anymore, as explained in the next section). While this works for him, it might not work for you, so please check with your doctor first.

How Christensen Discovered Vitamins C and E & Stopped Sneezing

Beginning when he was a teenager (back when the Earth was still cooling), co-author Christensen suffered from back-to-back colds and sinus infections, ailments not conducive to quality martial arts training sessions. He continued to suffer from frequent colds until about 10 years ago, when one day he read about the powerful anti-oxidant properties of combining vitamins C and E. After experimenting for a few months, he hit upon a combination of 600 mg. of vitamin E and 1,000 to 1,500 mg. of vitamin C spread over three doses during the day. Today, he catches a cold no more than once every 12 to 18 months.

Now, this is in no way scientific and shouldn't be construed as such. There may be other factors involved, though Christensen is adamant when he says there isn't. Will this regimen work for you? Who knows? As mentioned earlier, we encourage you to seek out a registered dietitian or doctor specializing in sports nutrition.

More Facts about Vitamins to Save You Money

Natural vitamins tend to be expensive since it's so pricey to extract them from natural sources. The solution? Don't buy them. Most vitamins in supplements are actually synthetic, which is okay since natural and manufactured vitamins have identical chemical structures. In other words, natural is no better than synthetic. The one exception is vitamin E, which in its natural form, is only slightly better absorbed and used. For long-term use, natural vitamin E might be too expensive to justify the slight advantage.

Store name brands are likely to be identical to well-known name brands, only much lower in price. There are only a few manufacturers of vitamins and minerals, and all tableters use the same raw materials. In fact, many big companies manufacture the brands found in supermarkets as well as the expensive brand names. The primary difference between them is the ingredients used, such as sugar, coloring, preservatives and the material used to make the supplement a tablet or a capsule.

When it comes to quality control, the big brand names generally score better than some small manufacturers, which of course you pay for at the register. It's worth it, though, because products from some small companies have been known to contain contaminants due to inferior production standards.

?

Confusion Over Daily Intake

So, how much of each vitamin and mineral should you take everyday? Should you take higher dosages because you workout regularly? The answers to these questions are…well, there doesn't seem to be an agreed upon answer to either question.

The United States Recommended Daily Allowance (USRDA), which was established about 50 years ago, lists one amount, while a new guideline called Reference Daily Intake (RDI) recommends another. A host of other lists compound the confusion, some recommending higher dosages than the USRDA and RDI, and others recommending lower amounts. Some nutritionists argue that athletes need more than sedentary folks, but other experts say there is no evidence of this. So what is a person to do?

It's in your best interest to talk to a qualified nutritionist, sports medicine specialist or doctor as to your needs (though not all doctors in general practice are knowledgeable about nutrition). It's also a good idea to have regular blood samples taken to determine if you are lacking in one or more vitamins or minerals.

Vitamins and minerals made without sugar or starch offer no advantage over those that do, but they often cost more. Just to be annoying, ask the clerk why you should pay more for something that isn't there, especially since it's not harmful when it is.

How Should Vitamins be Stored?

It's important to keep vitamins and minerals in a dark, cool place to prevent them from "spoiling," like apples in a bowl. It's best to store them in the refrigerator, and always keep the lids on the containers. A few grains of rice in the jar help prevent moisture from getting into the tablets. Think about buying a month's supply of a particular supplement, a two-month supply at the most. Those big jars of 500 are going to lose their freshness long before you swallow the last tablet.

When to Take Your Vitamins

The best time to take vitamins is during the day, after a meal. Never take them on an empty stomach because you just urinate them out and they might upset your tummy. This is especially true for the B and C vitamins that dissolve in water. Most experts say that it's best to take B vitamins in the morning because though they help calm your nerves, they often cause sleeplessness when taken at night.

Minerals

Twenty-two different minerals make up around five percent of your body weight, and every atom of each one existed in the rocks when the earth was formed over five billion years ago. You get minerals from the water you drink, water that once trickled through rocks, and you get them from the veggies and animals you eat that have been nourished from mineral-rich soil. These prehistoric metals work wondrously complex and vital miracles in your body that enable you to train healthily by balancing your body fluid levels, controlling your muscle contractions, carrying oxygen to your working muscles, and regulating your energy metabolism.

As with vitamins, the best way to get minerals is by eating a variety of natural foods, such as whole grain breads and cereals, lots of fresh fruits, deeply colored vegetables, lean meats, and low-fat dairy products. If your diet is balanced with the right amount of carbohydrates, proteins, and fats (roughly 40, 30 and 30), and at least 1,800 calories, most likely you are doing a good job getting the right amount of minerals.

While all minerals are needed for optimum health and continual success in training, let's take a quick look at three that are especially important to ensuring that you have sufficient energy for your martial arts — magnesium, chromium and zinc. Don't read into this that you should take mega doses, but rather just make sure you are getting your daily requirement. Likewise don't misread this as saying minerals give you energy, because they don't. Their critical role is to assist in its production.

Magnesium

Magnesium plays a critical role in your endurance. It exists mainly in your muscles and bones, where it assists with muscle contractions and energy metabolism. Studies with lab animals and real live people show that a deficiency in magnesium reduces endurance, and that low blood levels of magnesium are associated with decreased aerobic capacity. A low level of circulating magnesium has been seen in runners after completing a marathon, probably a result from mineral loss via sweating. If you have been working hard to improve your aerobic capacity but after 10 minutes of sparring you pant so hard you fog up your opponent's glasses, see if you are getting enough magnesium. The solution might be a simple adjustment in your diet and the addition of a mineral tablet.

Remember, more doesn't mean better. Since over supplementation can cause diarrhea and interfere with calcium absorption and metabolism, try to get your magnesium from food sources, such as nuts, molasses, whole grains and dark green, leafy vegetables, as opposed to taking a mega pill.

Calcium and Magnesium for the Female Fighter

As a female fighter, you might already know that it's especially important for you to get sufficient calcium, but you might be unaware that your body requires magnesium with it. Since your body works hard to keep the two minerals in balance, increasing one without increasing the other has little benefit.

Most sources say that you should consume 1,000 milligrams of each per day, more as you age. After menopause, for example, the recommended daily allowance is 1,500 milligrams of each. Recent research shows that pregnant women need to increase their intake to 1,500 to 2,000 mg per day. (No more full-contact sparring either.)

Insufficient calcium intake can result in your body "leeching" what it needs from your bones, thus weakening your skeletal system and putting you at risk of osteoporosis, or "brittle bones." Even a light fall or impact can leave you with breaks. Since you are in the business of kicking and punching bags and bodies, brittle bones are not what you want.

By the way, smoking, excessive alcohol consumption and a regular diet of fast food all contribute to loss of calcium. The anecdote is to avoid these things, train hard (exercise strengthens your skeletal system) and monitor your daily intake of these two critical minerals. [15][16]

Chromium

Some nutritionists, especially those who sell the stuff, claim that chromium burns body fat while it builds muscle. This is why chromium picolinate has become the supplement of choice for so many runners, bodybuilders, martial artists and dieters. Co-author Christensen got on the bandwagon in the late 1980s and found that the only thing he lost after four months taking the stuff was the money in his wallet. Recent studies concur that chromium picolinate won't melt even a little fat from your body.

While the mineral doesn't fulfill our fantasy of a fat-burning and muscle-building mineral, chromium is still vitally important to your punching and kicking. It assists the hormone insulin in processing carbohydrates, which you know is your number one source for energy. Research on endurance athletes has shown that exercise speeds chromium loss through the urine following exercise. This has led some researchers to believe that endurance athletes need more chromium, particularly since they tend to eat a high-carbohydrate diet that requires more insulin (hence more chromium) for carbohydrate processing.

Chromium is a bit of a problem child because scientists don't have enough hard information yet to firmly establish an RDA. It's a difficult mineral to measure in foods, and scientists can't figure out how to track whether we are getting enough. They do know that there is a range of 50 to 200 micrograms that is considered safe and adequate. No doubt you get that much now, unless you eat a lot junk food, such as donuts, cakes and other sweets. These bad foods are low in chromium while at the same time boosting your need for it to help process the carbs.

As with magnesium, it's best to get this mineral from food sources rather than from a supplement. Getting too much chromium, which could only happen if you pop chromium supplements, can hamper your absorption of iron and zinc. Some chromium-rich foods are wheat germ, nuts and — *tuh-duh!* — beer! It's true. Aren't you glad you bought this book? But you got to be of age.

Zinc

Although zinc is critical to your body, you don't need a lot of it since a little goes a long way. You have about two grams in your body that works in tandem with more than 100 different enzymes, many of which participate in that all-important process — energy metabolism.

Zinc is also essential for a healthy immune system. Endurance exercise seems to reduce zinc levels in the body, which may be part of the reason why some endurance athletes are more prone to colds and upper respiratory tract infections immediately following races or tough workouts. In one study, athletes lost twice as much zinc through their urine following a six-mile run compared to when they didn't exercise. Since a small amount of zinc is lost in sweat, and many people don't get their RDA to begin with, it's clear why up to 40 percent of athletes may have below-normal levels of zinc in their blood.

Men need 15 milligrams of zinc and women need 12. Unfortunately, the best sources of it are found in relatively high-fat food, such as oysters, clams, liver and several other meats. If these turn you off, you can also get zinc from low-fat foods like wheat germ, fortified breakfast cereals and black-eyed peas. Know that over supplementing with zinc has been shown to lower the "good" HDL cholesterol and raise "bad" LDL cholesterol.

Macro and Trace Minerals

Minerals are broken down into two kinds: macrominerals and trace minerals. Macro means "large" in Greek and your body needs larger amounts of macrominerals than trace minerals. The macromineral group is made up of calcium, phosphorous, magnesium, sodium, potassium, chloride, and sulfur

Though your body needs trace minerals, it needs just a tiny amount of each. Trace minerals are chromium, cobalt, copper, fluoride, iodine, iron, manganese, molybdenum, nickel, selenium, silicon, tin, vanadium, and zinc. Scientists still don't know how much of these you need each day.

Too Much of a Good Thing

If you eat healthily, meaning you are getting lots of minerals through your food, including foods fortified with 50 to 100 percent of the RDA of minerals, and you take a mineral supplement, you just might be taking in too much, the impact of which nutrition professionals don't yet fully understand. Overdoing it might lead to a mineral imbalance or toxicity. If you live by the code "if a little bit is good, then more must be better," know that it's dangerous when following the code with mineral supplements. This is because more of one mineral may prevent your system from absorbing another. This can occur when different ones compete for pathways through your body or when they interact with each other and form a mineral complex that is poorly absorbed. You might not feel the effects right away, but scientists believe taking high doses might create future health problems.

The key to mineral intake is to stay in balance. The best way to do this is to eat a well-balanced diet and—if you think you might be deficient in a mineral—talk to your doctor or registered dietitian. [17][18]

Iron: Women and Men

Due to their menstrual cycle, women need a sufficient intake of iron to help rebuild red blood cells. Failure to do so can lead to iron deficiency or, in extreme cases, anemia. This is not good for any woman, and it's especially bad for the female martial artist since a diet low in iron can limit the amount of oxygen the blood carries, meaning physical performance will be severely impaired. Other problems associated with iron deficiency are a weakened immune system, irritability, poor learning ability and a shortened attention span.

Female fighters can avoid all this by getting between 12 and 18 milligrams of iron per day. That is a wide range so it's vital to check with your doctor to pinpoint your needs.

It's uncommon for men to suffer iron deficiency and they should not supplement with it except under doctor's orders. Generally, they need about seven milligrams. Men who take more are at risk for heart and liver problems.

Teenagers need 10-13 mg per day. [19] [20]

Fast Facts

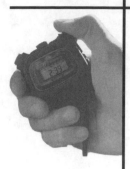

- Although water doesn't contain even one lonesome calorie, it's still the most important and critical of all nutrients.

- If you don't drink liquids to replace what is lost, your blood becomes concentrated, meaning that it thickens and puts a tremendous strain on your heart.

- Studies show that sweating five percent of your water can affect your performance up to 30 percent.

- Thirst is not always an indicator of dehydration.

- Divide your bodyweight in half. Your answer is the number of ounces of water you should be drinking each day for maintenance.

- Some experts say you need sports drinks for their added mineral content and quick absorption rate, especially if you train at an intense level for at least 30 minutes or at a moderate level for one hour or more.

- Any time you train at a low intensity for less than half an hour, fortified sports drinks are a waste of money, since the sodium you get in your normal diet is all you need.

- Caffeine "loosens up" your body's fat, which can be used for energy during a workout.

- One glass of alcohol has at least 100 to125 calories. Drink three glasses a day and you add a pound of fat every 12 days or so.

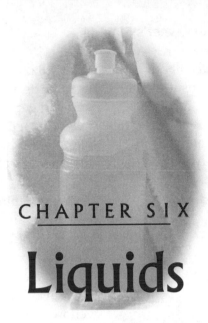

CHAPTER SIX

Liquids

Since roughly 70 percent of your body weight is water, it makes sense that you carefully manage your intake to stay hydrated throughout the day. It's important even for people leading sedentary lives, like couch potatoes and desk jockeys, but for martial artists who push their bodies through rigorous training regimens, taking in sufficient liquid can mean the difference between peak performance and poor performance, good health and poor health, and even life and death. Although water doesn't contain even one lonesome calorie, it's still the most important and critical of all nutrients. You can stagger around a blazing desert for days without food, but go more than two or three days without water and you end up as cactus fertilizer.

When You Don't Drink Enough

To put into perspective how vital it is that you continuously sip water as you train, here is an example of just one problem caused by a lack of hydration. Say you weigh 150 pounds and during a tough sparring session you sweat out more than two percent of your bodyweight, a typical amount. A two percent loss equals three pounds of water, a quart and a half. While this might not sound significant, it is. Worse case scenario: If you don't do some slurping to replace the loss, your blood becomes concentrated, meaning that it thickens and puts a tremendous strain on your heart. Thick blood can clot, which isn't a good thing if you plan on having another birthday. The least of your problems is that you have less blood plasma, which brings on fatigue quickly as your body struggles to carry oxygenated blood throughout your system.

There is nothing complicated about drinking water other than ensuring that you get enough, even when not thirsty. In fact, a lack of thirst can be a sign your body is in desparate need of hydration. Let's look closer as to why you need to drink sufficient water before, during and after your training and what happens when you don't.

Dehydration

Dehydration occurs when the body's water level drops below that required for adequate circulation and normal body function, and it can zap you in as little as 30 minutes after you begin training, especially in hot weather. Before you can say, "Ugh, I feel strange," you are at risk of heat exhaustion or heat stroke, which kills over 400 people a year.

Symptoms

Keep this important fact in the forefront of your mind: Thirst is not always an indicator of dehydration. If you aren't taking in water every 15 to 20 minutes during hard training, you might move into an early stage of dehydration without knowing it. As it becomes more pronounced, your face flushes, your thirst becomes extreme and, the two biggees, you might stop sweating and your skin turns cold and dry. Then comes an inability to urinate, or if you do, it's dark yellow. Then you grow

weak, dizzy, your muscles cramp, your head hurts, your get saliva gets thick, and you get sleepy. It's then that the tall, skinny, pale-faced man in the long black overcoat - the old coffin maker — measures you for size.

There is nothing in any of these stages that you want; the good news is that it's easy to avoid them by simply drinking water on a regular basis (don't you wish all problems were as easy to correct?). If you have thirst, dry mouth and dark yellow urine, you need to immediately drink at least a quart of water. If you have severe symptoms, such as muscle cramps, weakness, or dizziness, take at least a 15-minute break to drink as much fluid as you can handle. It might even be a good idea to quit training for the day.

Instructors Who Don't Allow Students to Drink

During prolonged sparring, kata practice or drills, water is lost through your sweat at an hourly rate 285 times greater than you lose when watching the boob tube lying on your sofa. Even jogging at a comfortable training pace for 60 minutes can drain up to two quarts of water from your body. If you don't do some serious sipping to replace the loss, your performance suffers as will your body.

Many good but uninformed instructors don't allow their students to drink during class - this is wrong, and you can quote us. If that offends some instructors, sorry, but there is no argument with this. If your instructor prohibits students from drinking water, we strongly suggest that you respectfully discuss the matter with him, or perhaps ask for a class meeting where you can talk about the material in this book or information you have on water from any other source.

If his reasoning is based on not wanting his class disrupted for drinks, ask if you can brainstorm ways students can take a quick swig without causing a problem (students in our classes keep their water bottles along the wall and have a drink whenever they want, taking no longer than 15 seconds). If he prohibits drinking water because of a custom founded by an ancient master (one unenlightened as to the importance of hydration), ask if he can enforce discipline some other way that isn't hazardous to his students' health. If he still holds fast to his way, remind him how expensive lawsuits are should one of his students collapse.

If your instructor says he is going to continue his old ways because he doesn't believe the information, you have to wonder in what other areas of fitness, health and modern training methods he is lacking knowledge. You might even consider whether you want to to continue under his guidance. Yes, it's that serious.

One uninformed instructor One of co-author Demeere's first instructors believed in teaching strict discipline, courage and perseverance through harsh methods that were used on him when he was a student. He made his followers do hundreds of push-ups each class, forms, sparring, drills, and forced them to stand in a low horse stance while hitting them with sticks. There were never water breaks though sweating was profuse, especially during the summer. When class was over, Demeere says he would drink two or three beverages, sportsdrinks or softdrinks (the instructor's no-drinking policy made the school's bar owner wealthy), and when he got home, he drank a bottle of water or milk, usually in one gulp. When he left that instructor and began training with one that allowed water breaks, his performance improved dramatically. Today, he carries a bottle of water with him all day and downs another full one during training.

Sweating

Your body functions normally between 97.7 and 99.5 degrees. When you kick and punch, it generates more heat, necessitating that you sweat to release some of it and to prevent your internal temperature from rising to a dangerously high level, called hyperthermia. Hypothermia is just the opposite, a condition where your body temperature drops too low: 95 degrees is considered mild hypothermia and 80 degrees is considered severe, near death. Your body needs to function in that narrow margin of 97.7 to 99.5, so that all your body functions work correctly.

When you spar for five rounds or do a form 10 times in a row, your body heats up quickly so that in just minutes you are sweating like a 7th grader waiting to see the principal. To avoid health problems and keep your performance at its optimum, you must replace the lost water. Studies show that sweating five percent of your water can affect your performance up to 30 percent.

For a visual, here are two easy equations:

No water = poor health = poor performance

Water = good health = good performance

Questions, class?

How Much Water and How Often

Let's look at ways to determine the quantity you need and when you should pour it down your gullet. It's easy to determine how much you get when you drink from an eight-ounce glass or a 32-ounce water bottle. To determine your intake from a drinking fountain, you have to count your gulps. One gulp is one ounce for most adults with average-sized mouths (some mothers-in-law have been known to take in a quart with one gulp). When training, take six gulps about every 20 minutes.

Nontraining days   It's common now to see everyone from construction workers to downtown executives toting a bottle of water. This is a good thing, as it indicates that more and more people are getting educated as to the importance of staying hydrated. There is still confusion, however, as to how much one should drink. "I drink two gallons a day," we have heard people brag. Others say they try to get a quart down in the morning and another in the afternoon. A few try to play catch-up at the end of the day and drink eight glasses at once. None of these methods are accurate or particularly good for you. Here is an easy formula to help you take the guesswork out of it.

Divide your bodyweight in half. *Tu-duh!* Your answer is the number of ounces of water you should be drinking each day for maintenance. Here is how it looks if you are a 200-pound brute:

200 lbs divided by 2 = 100 ounces of water (not 100 pounds of water)

So, if you drink your water from an eight-ounce glass, you need to knock back about 12 of them a day. If you drink from a 32-ounce quart bottle, you need three full ones each day for optimum health. Don't drink your entire daily requirement at breakfast but ration it throughout the day (did we really have to tell you that?).

Training days   On training days, you need to factor in your sweating. An easy way to determine how much additional water you need beyond what you need for optimum health is to weigh yourself before and after your workout. The difference on the scale is what you lost sweating. You need 16 ounces of water for every pound lost. Tip: Don't weigh yourself wearing a uniform that has soaked up your sweat. Strip down to a grin and weigh yourself before and after training. Here is the formula if you weigh 200 pounds:

198 lbs. after training   (2 lbs. lost through sweating)

2 lbs. = 32 ounces of additional water

100 ounces (nontraining day requirement) + 32 ounces = 132 ounces for the day

You can replace your two-pound loss with four, 8-ounce glasses of water or an extra quart from your water bottle.

Before training   To supply your body with a good amount of hydration for your training, drink two to three eight-ounce glasses of water about two hours before your session and then another glass or two about 15 or 20 minutes just before it starts. Once training begins, drink about six ounces every 15 to 20 minutes, and take in another glass or two afterwards, more if you feel you need it. Should you fail to drink water two hours before class but then drink a bottle just as it starts, it won't do you as much good since it takes time to fully absorb the liquid into your system. It can also cause your tummy to bloat so that your training partner thinks he is working with a pregnant person.

Consider all factors   Since no two classes are the same, your water requirements will vary. Factors such as room temperature, humidity, clothing, and altitude all influence your needs.

It's also important to consider the intensity of the class. One in which you spar, do lots of hard reps or perform your 100-movement kata over and over requires that you take in more water than during a class geared toward performing new techniques slowly and methodically.

Don't go by thirst   Take your sips on a schedule, rather than waiting until you are thirsty. Remember, by the time you feel thirst, you are already lacking vital fluids, and your performance is probably beginning to deteriorate. Since it takes a while for that gulp of fluid to get into your system, you won't benefit from it right away. This is why it's best to take sips routinely every 15 to 20 minutes.

Are Sports Drinks Good for Fighters?

Many athletes have been drafted to star in commercials promoting various sports drinks (actually, they are paid a lot of money), in an effort to make you believe that you too need these drinks to perform like these elite sports figures. Well, you might or you might not, because it depends on lots of other things, too, like how you train, eat, sleep and think. Let's take a quick look at sports drinks and see what they have to offer you and your martial arts training. We won't talk brand names, since there are over 100-plus drinks on the market, but we will provide you with information as to how to read labels.

When you sweat profusely, you lose water as well as sodium, potassium, calcium, magnesium, chloride, bicarbonate, phosphate and sulphate. Sodium loss is critical (to see how much is lost through sweating, get one of your more nervous buddies to lift his arm and count the salt rings on his shirt), as it helps regulate fluid balance and plays a vital role in muscle contractions. Can you imagine kicking a heavy bag without your muscles contracting? It would be like whipping the bag with a limp noodle.

Several years before he learned the importance of hydration, co-author Christensen tested a student for black belt, a four-hour exam with no rest and little water. Twice the student asked for permission to sip water and both times Christensen and the examiners nodded, but with frowns of disapproval. Near the end of the test, the student begged for and was given permission to use the restroom so that he could vomit. Shortly after that, his abdominal muscles contracted so hard that they forced him to bend forward. Still the test went on, though the student could no longer stand straight. When it finally concluded, he had to be driven to Christensen's home where he collapsed on the floor in a fetal position. It took two mineral tablets and countless glasses of water before he could uncurl himself and sit up.

Due to Christensen's ignorance as to the value of hydration, he could have caused his student grave health risks, especially if the test had gone much longer. Oh yes, he passed and is today a third-degree black. His teacher has apologized several times over the years for his ignorance.

Christensen attributes the mineral tablets — especially the sodium — as helping his student recover from his dangerous depletion. Today, many sports drinks are enriched with minerals that replace those depleted in hard training. Some of the better ones even have a small percentage of carbohydrates, which speeds up the absorption of the water.

Whether you need to spend your allowance on sports drinks depends on the severity of your training. Some experts say you need them for their added mineral content and quick absorption rate, especially if you train at an intense level for at least 30 minutes or at a moderate level for one hour or more. However, any time you train at a low intensity for less than half an hour, fortified sports drinks are a waste of money, since the sodium you get in your normal diet is all you need. Also, if you drank enough water before you begin training (as mentioned earlier), a 30-minute workout isn't long enough for your performance to be affected by lost fluids. Of course you can still have a sports drink to benefit from the liquid, just as you benefit from water.

How do you train?   A typically hard karate, kickboxing, taekwondo, and kung fu class, a hard grappling class, such as judo, jiu-jitsu and wrestling, and a mixed arts class, such as vale tudo and pancrase are generally intense enough to warrant the use of sports drinks. Usually, the softer arts, such as tai chi chuan or aikido, don't fit into this category, unless the students are practicing hard and fast self-defense applications. Now, if you want to drink sports drinks, though you aren't training hard, you won't gain anything and you probably won't hurt anything, though you will get extra calories and expensive urine.

Speaking of calories Check the label to see how many carbs are floating in your sports drink. If it contains over eight percent, you might experience the dreaded energy spike, followed by a pronounced drop in energy soon after. Some experts say that sports drinks over seven percent take longer to get into the system, which defeats their purpose of keeping you hydrated during physical activities. None of these negatives are good when you still have half a class left or you want to enter more than one division at a tournament.

We stongly suggest that you experiment carefully with the different brands of sports drinks and quantities to see which ones are best for you. Don't wait until the day of a competition to try a new drink.

Facts about Sports Drinks

- Choose sports drinks that contain 14 to 19 grams of carbs, which equal 6 to 8 percent carbs, and 50 to 80 calories per eight-ounce serving. The carbs help increase the rate of absorption and delay the onset of fatigue in an especially long training session.

- Sports drinks with greater than 10% sugar solution are too high in carbs, resulting in slow absorption, nausea, cramps or diarrhea. Less fluid absorption means greater risk of dehydration and a higher body temperature, which adds up to poor performance and stress on your health.

- Choose sports drinks that contain glucose, glucose polymers, moltodextrin or sucrose as the carbohydrate source. Sucrose and glucose have been proven effective in delivering energy and hastening the rate of fluid absorption.

- Since you don't sweat out vitamins don't buy drinks with added vitamins .

- Drink between eight and 24 ounces of a sports beverage two hours before you train or compete, and drink another eight ounces fifteen minutes before your activity.

- During your training or competition, drink six ounces of your sports drink every 15 to 20 minutes.

- Drink at least 16 ounces of fluid for every pound lost during your session.

Water Intoxication

Yes, you can get too much water, but it's not the kind of intoxication where you dance on a table top and swing your shirt over your head. It's a problem usually associated with long distance running and cycling events, though it's conceivable it could happen at a vigorous all-day tournament or seminar. Water intoxication, or hyponatremia, was reported in nearly one out of five marathon runners and more than one out of four finishers in the Hawaiian Ironman Triathlon in studies reported in *Medicine and Science in Sports & Exercise*, respectively. [21]

How it Happens

Drinking excessive amounts of water during a lengthy and strenuous event dilutes the salt content of the liquid part of your blood (blood plasma). Since you are already losing salt through sweating, drinking excessive amounts of water drastically reduces the salt needed by your brain, heart and muscles. Ironically, the symptoms of water intoxication are similar to the symptoms of dehydration: nausea, fatigue, and reduced thinking ability.

Definition of a bad day   You are at an all-day seminar where a competitor, who has not read this book, is slumped in the corner suffering dehydration symptoms from going all day without drinking. You are slumped next to him but suffering from water intoxication symptoms because you drank too much (you read the book but skipped this section). The medics first treat the other fighter by pouring a quart of water down his dry throat. Thinking you are also dehydrated because your symptoms are the same, and that you are protesting because you are delirious, they force you to drink a quart of water, too.

How Much is Enough?

The water requirement for most hard fighting martial artists is eight to 16 ounces per hour. Yes, this is a wide range, but it's difficult to nail an exact amount as it depends on individual sweating rates, body size, room temperature, training intensity and so on. The wide range isn't limited to the martial arts. Runners, for example, are also told to drink between eight and 18 ounces of water, while soccer players are instructed to drink five to 12 ounces.

As is often the case, you need to experiment to see what is best for you. As mentioned previously, weigh yourself before and after your training. If you gained weight, you know you drank more than you needed.

Before we move on to carbonated drinks, alcohol and coffee, here is a recap on water and sports drinks:

• Never restrict fluids during exercise.

• Drink water, diluted fruit juice or diluted sports drink during exercise, practice and competition.

- During exercise, drink about four to six ounces of fluid every 15 to 20 minutes. Cold drinks are absorbed more rapidly.

- If you exercise vigorously for less than 30 minutes you don't need a sports drink, as water will suffice. If you exercise strenuously for more than one hour, or moderately for more than two hours, you might benefit from an energy drink. Be sure the carbohydrate content doesn't exceed seven percent by weight. A higher percentage slows absorption and may cause stomach cramps.

- Avoid drinks with caffeine or alcohol that dehydrate you (more on this next).

- Always make fluids a part of your exercise routine.

Carbonated Drinks

Carbonated drinks are a poor choice before, during or after your training or competing because you run the risk of getting stomach cramps and an energy spike followed by a drop in energy. Oh yes, carbonated drinks make some people belch, which is a little tacky when performing kata.

Alcohol: Yes or No?

Picture a drunken, obnoxious black belt leaning against the bar, clutching a pitcher of beer and bragging to his buddies about his deadly skills. He is so full of beer and himself that he doesn't even notice the giggles and laughter of those around him, people convinced that the martial arts turn people into fools. Fiction? No. Sadly, it happens often.

Unless you are starring with Jackie Chan in the next *Drunken Master* movie and doing research by getting intoxicated and fighting, there is nothing in alcohol that you need. You definitely don't need it when competing regularly in tournaments or preparing for your next belt exam, and you definitely don't need it when trying to lose a few pounds. Here are a few more reasons to avoid alcohol or, at the most, use it in moderation:

- Alcohol causes excessive urination. If you drink two beers before training — heaven forbid! — and then sweat heavily during your workout, you risk dehydration, fatigue, weakness, and dizziness, while placing undue stress on your kidneys.

- Alcohol produces a beer belly. Although a gram of alcohol contains only seven calories, they are empty ones, meaning they can't be stored in your muscles for energy. When that beer, wine or whiskey sour hits your stomach, your body considers the alcohol a toxin, and to clear it out quickly, it puts the metabolizing of carbs, protein and fats on standby, and slows many of your body's other vital functions.

- Alcohol causes energy spikes and energy downers as a result of how your body is forced to metabolize your carbs.

- Alcohol suppresses your central nervous system. A drunk has poor balance, poor control of his body, and poor eye and hand coordination. Obviously, this isn't a good thing for a fighter in training. If there is anything good about having a suppressed central nervous system it's that you feel less pain should you get into a real fight and your assailant beats you to oblivion. Of course, after you sober up in the hospital, it's going to hurt a lot.

- Alcohol is a drug; it's addictive. Alcoholism has serious short- and long-term effects on your life in every area: social, family, financial, health and work. There is no way you can be a successful martial artist when your life is falling apart from alcohol addiction.

- Your liver hates the stuff. Drink excessively and this all-important organ goes into overdrive to keep up. Most alcoholics' livers are shot, which isn't a good thing because they are good to have.

Your Authors Have an Occasional Sip

Now, your authors are not teetotalers; we appreciate a good beer or glass of wine. However, we never drink an entire six-pack at a time or a bottle of wine at one sitting. We savor and enjoy one glass, on rare occasions, two.

Co-author Demeere wasn't always so strict. Living in Belgium where he is convinced they have the best beer in the world (co-author Christensen argues that Oregon has the best microbrews in the world), he says that beer was always around when he was growing up. There isn't even an enforced age limit since it's just considered part of the fabric of Belgian society.

Demeere was already drinking regularly before he began training in the martial arts. Since he had a fast metabolism, made even faster by his daily training, it took but one glass to intoxicate him, much to the delight of his friends. By the time he was 18, he had become a serious martial arts competitor, and was no longer drinking the way he had when younger. When his friends complained about his sobriety, saying he wasn't as fun as he used to be, Demeere just shrugged off their taunts, as the martial arts had given him the confidence to resist peer pressure. The realization that he didn't need alcohol to have a good time, combined with his increased training and competition, made beer a rare indulgence.

He is retired now, though he still trains hard, and has a beer only on rare occasions.

Is Alcohol Healthy?

There have been numerous studies done about the health benefits of drinking a glass or two of alcohol. They show that alcohol raises the level of HDL, the so-called "good cholesterol," which protects against fatty blockage in the arteries and inhibits blood clotting. But before you get too giddy, know that these findings have recently come under fire. Too many people used the information as an excuse to drink more, in some cases, a lot more. Unfortunately for them, they should have read the studies further: The findings were seen only in people who drank less than one or two drinks a day; when they had more the benefits disappeared.

One study placed the correlation between improved cardiovascular health and drinking a glass of wine on other factors. For example, it found that many people who drink wine come from a slightly higher social status than those who don't drink it or who drink other alcoholic beverages. They found that wine drinkers are more inclined to take care of themselves and have access to better medical services. The study didn't say that wine is completely without benefit, but it shows another side to the findings.

Last call We suggest that you approach alcohol conservatively and

that you never drink it if you are under the legal age. Stay away from it completely if you are training for a competition or belt test, and if you are trying to drop some pounds, know that alcohol is brimming with calories. One glass has 100 to125 of the little buggers. Drink three glasses a day and you add a pound of fat every 12 days or so.

Coffee

In *Fighter's Fact Book*, Christensen wrote "Will coffee help your karate training? Maybe, but you need to decide if it's worth it. I have used coffee for years to get a slight boost in energy for my workouts without harmful side effects. Other people, however, have problems since caffeine can make one's blood sugar level fluctuate, and because it contains acid, it can cause heartburn and stomach problems during training. But not everyone experiences these problems. If you do, you have to decide if the energy kick is worth it.

"In a study at Ball University, several athletes drank coffee without knowing it (how did they do that?), and every one of them found that their performance improved considerably; in particular, they were able to exercise seven percent longer than without coffee. In another study published in the International Journal of Sports Nutrition, one group of athletes was given a placebo of glucose, and another group was given six mg. of caffeine per two pounds of each person's bodyweight. They were then tested as they cycled at different speeds. The end result showed that the caffeine group performed significantly better than the group that consumed glucose."

While all of the above is still valid, new data continues to come out about America's favorite beverage and, happily for all of us caffeine connoisseurs, it's not all bad. Actually, some of the findings are good. So pour yourself a cup and read on.

We know that coffee can cause anxiety, miscarriages, insomnia, dehydration, and other health problems, which has caused some health organizations to ask the Food and Drug Administration (FDA) to require food makers to label the caffeine content of foods and drinks. They think we should know how much extra caffeine we are getting in our teas, candy bars, headache pills, sodas and a myriad of other products.

We don't have an argument with this, especially since many people have a low tolerance for caffeine and may be risking their health by consuming too much, or at the least, giving themselves miserable days because of inadvertent excessive consumption.

If you drink coffee and suffer regularly from upset stomach, jitters, diarrhea, insomnia and so on, we strongly suggest you take a hard look at how much you drink and when you drink it, and then talk to your doctor about the problem. Although we are talking here about the benefits of coffee for your training, you and the doctor may decide it's not worth your health and quality of life.

Nutritionists, the FDA and others who study such things are continuously coming out with new data. The preponderance of it is good news for hard training martial artists, though you still need to tread with caution, keeping in mind what the old white-bearded sage says about eating, drinking, and everything else you do in your life: "Everything in moderation." (He is starting to be a real killjoy.)

Understand that as we talk about how to use coffee to give you a training boost, we are talking about a simple mug of joe, your father's coffee, not one of those space-age double caramel, triple chocolate, triple cream, with brownie chunks, five tablespoons of sugar and a scoop of ice cream in a 32-ounce container (we just made this up but it sounds great, doesn't it?) totaling 1,250 calories. No, we are talking about a basic, old fashion cup of coffee, one that doesn't have one calorie.

Mental Benefits

Every student pulling an all-night study fest, every droopy-eyed nightshift worker and every person needing a first-thing-in-the-morning jumpstart knows the value of coffee as a wake-me-up. It's universally used to increase alertness, provide clearer thinking, increase the ability to concentrate for long periods, and just basically dissolve those brain "fuzzies." According to one British study published in the journal *Physiology & Behavior*, 1999, test takers who drank caffeineated coffee could process new information and fight fatigue better than those who had the decaffeinated drink. It didn't improve their memories, though.

Say you are having a day when your brain is tired, sleepy or, for whatever reason, you just feel dumb as a brick, and now you are on your way to a complicated kata session, an intricate tai chi class or a stick fighting class in which you are learning complex patterns. A cup or two of coffee might be the nudge you need to more clearly understand the teaching. You might also find, as some competitors have, that it stimulates the brain to help them get psyched before a tournament. Now, if you haven't used coffee for this purpose, you should first experiment during a training session to know that it works for you. It's never a good idea to try something for the first time on competition day.

Training Benefits

Though there have been few studies, there are tons of anecdotal evidence to show that coffee provides a bump of energy to help you get a little better workout than you would have had without it. At this writing, there are all kinds of theories as to how it gives you that bump, but no absolutes. There are arguments that coffee allows for increased fat utilization, arguments that it increases blood glucose, and arguments that the liver glycogen is broken down faster and manufactured faster. Some say the bump comes from a

combination of all of these. For our purposes here, we aren't going to elaborate on all the technical possibilities. We are just going take another sip and say that if the technical aspect is of interest to you, then take it upon yourself to research the findings that continue to come out.

If you haven't developed a tolerance to coffee, which happens to people who drink large amounts daily, caffeine will probably provide a boost for your workout or competition. This is why the International Olympic Committee limits its use by competitors. The Committee allows athletes to show no more than 12 mcg of caffeine in a milliliter of urine, which you get from 800 mg caffeine, or six to eight cups of coffee, in an hour or two.

An Unpleasant Image

Here is a bit of trivia we found in our research that you might find unpleasant to think about. Just before the 1984 Olympics, the United States bicycling team was caught using caffeine suppositories (yipes!), each containing 3,000 milligrams of caffeine. Now, a regular cup of coffee contains only 100-150 milligrams, which is considerably lower than what the bikers were getting. The good news is that drinking a cup of coffee doesn't require as much bending and twisting to get into your system.

Although there are no known studies on caffeine consumption as it relates to martial arts performance in training and competition, there have been studies on such endurance athletes as runners, swimmers, rowers and bicyclists. They found out that there is a marked improvement when coffee is consumed before an event. (We could have told them that and saved them thousands of dollars.)

Study on endurance athletes In a study conducted at McMaster University in Ontario, researchers gave either a placebo or about 600 milligrams of caffeine (approximately the amount in four cups of brewed coffee) to five endurance athletes before they rode to exhaustion on exercise bicycles. The study was carried out in a randomized, double-blind fashion (athletes who initially ingested caffeine tried the placebo at a later date and vice versa; neither athletes nor researchers were initially aware of who was actually taking in caffeine). After they could no longer ride, the scientists used an electrical device to stimulate muscles in the lower portions of the exhausted athletes' legs. When the electrical stimulation was greatest, the 'caffeine-loaded' muscles proved to be about 25 percent stronger (meaning they contracted about 25 percent more forcefully with caffeine than with placebo). [22]

Study on short-term high intensity workouts One group of swimmers was given coffee, .6 mg x kilograms of bodyweight, and the other group a placebo before a swim trial lasting a little under 25 minutes. The group that swam on coffee had better times and a lower level of exhaustion after.

How Much?

Not as much as you might think. A 150-pound person requires less than a 225-pound brute, and a person who normally drinks one cup of coffee a day requires less than a person who drinks it throughout the day, since the frequent drinker most likely has developed a degree of tolerance to its effects. As we can't pinpoint exactly your needs, we can give you a range of 200 to 600 milligrams (one to four, 6-ounce cups). If four cups of coffee sounds like a lot, it is. How would you like to catch a sidekick in the stomach after downing four mugs full?

Over the years we have seen outstanding results on students and on ourselves after drinking two cups about an hour before training. We extended the range to four cups here because some of the studies used that many. The question has to be asked: Is more than four cups better? No. Studies show that there is a saturation point where there is no longer a training effect after 600 milligrams.

How to Use It

It's not advisable to drink two to four cups of coffee every time you train, because it's quite easy to develop a tolerance. It's best to use caffeine as a pick-me-up only on those days when you absolutely need a nudge. The effects last roughly two to two-and-a-half hours, so it's important to give thought to timing your cups with your class or competition.

Warning: If you have high blood pressure, allergies, weak liver and other problems easily aggravated by the caffeine stimulant, you should not consume it at all, let alone use it as a preworkout nudge. Also, know that coffee is a diuretic, meaning it makes you urinate more. The average person retains about half to two-thirds of the liquid in the coffee, tea or caffeineated soda; the rest is urinated out. Those who consume caffeineated beverages regularly retain even more liquid. [23] To make up for the loss, we suggest you drink an equal amount of water. For example, say tonight you want an energy bump from two cups of coffee before your workout. Go ahead, but be sure to make up for the water loss by drinking two extra cups of water.

We strongly encourage you to check with your doctor, and only after he gives you the okay should you include the occasional coffee before your workouts. Begin with one cup and monitor how you feel prior, during and after your training session. If you think you can handle more, add another cup. As we noted just above, it's our experience that two cups have been optimum for everyone we have worked with, though some studies report success with four cups.

If you feel nausea, dizziness, bad stomach and excessive jitters, immediately cut back on your consumption. If drinking less doesn't help, stop drinking it all together.

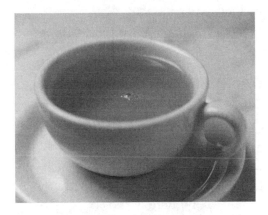

Green Tea

Green tea has been getting lots of press lately and that is a good thing. But will it help you throw a better roundhouse kick? Not directly. If you have a lousy kick today and you drink green tea for a week, well, your kick will still be lousy. Indirectly, though, green tea helps your quality of life so that you feel healthy enough to work extra hard to improve your roundhouse.

Green tea and black tea come from the same plant but green tea is less processed than black. Green tea increases your blood circulation, which is important for training energy and the overall health of your heart, and both green and black tea contain goodies that fight cancer, tooth decay, stomach problems, colds and more. Have you ever tried to punch the bag when you had an aching cavity or a nasty cold? Fewer colds and healthy teeth add up to better workouts (and a dazzling smile). New research has shown that the tea's antioxidants may help fight cataracts, at least in laboratory rats. The Chinese, who are among the world's heaviest tea drinkers, have a below-average incidence of cataracts.

What to Look for at the Store

Go the tea section of your neighborhood grocery and read the labels of three or four brands that offer green tea. Choose the one that has — are you ready for this?— polyphenols and/or Epigallocatechingallate, usually noted as EGCG. You want a tea that contains at least 40 to 50 percent of polyphenol and 10 to 16 percent of that big word, EGCG.

Some companies even sell these in capsule form, which are usually found in health food stores and the health food section of your grocery. If you want to drink it in tea form, there are several leading brands that contain both important ingredients. Most offer a caffeine-free tea, which is the best way for you to drink it, especially after training. Remember, caffeine is a diuretic and drains water from your body, something you don't want after having dripped sweat in class for a couple hours.

How Much?

Depending on which study you read, you should drink one to four cups a day. Co-author Christensen drinks one to three cups a day and feels that it has helped his overall health. Although green tea can be purchased cold in a can, at least one study showed that it should be consumed as a hot beverage.

Make a cup or two of green tea part of your daily ritual and enjoy these benefits:

• Strengthens your immune system

• Prevents cancer

• Prevents heart disease

• Prevents digestive disorders

• Reduces cholesterol levels

• Reduces blood pressure

• Prevents plaque, tooth decay cavities

• Keeps your skin healthy and youthful

Milk

The dairy industry encourages you to drink milk all day and walk around with that disgusting milk film on your upper lip for no other reason than they really care about your health. Or, could it be that they want you to buy their product so their executives can drive fancy cars and live in fancy houses, while you walk around with that milk smear on your face and your belly jiggling from all those milk calories? So, are we being caustic here because you shouldn't drink it? At the risk of being wishy-washy again: It depends.

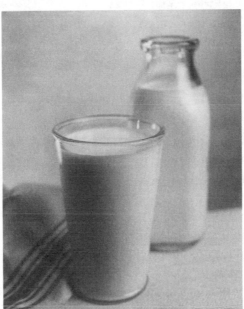

Whole Milk: The Bad

Though the dairy industry says it's an ideal food, a complete food and "it's good for every body," the truth is that many adults have a problem with some of the components found in it, especially whole milk. Three out of four people who don't originate from northern European ancestry don't have the enzyme lactase that breaks down milk sugar, lactose. This is commonly referred to as being lactose intolerant, a problem that causes such disgusting symptoms as gas, stomach cramping, bloating and diarrhea. Wait. It gets worse.

The protein in a glass of milk, called casein, is an irritant to many drinkers and is thought to play a role in causing allergies and stimulating mucus, thus leading to frequent colds, ear infections, bronchitis, asthma, eczema, sinus problems and even arthritis. Still think that milk stain on the upper lip looks cute? Consider this. The fat in whole milk is called butterfat, and it isn't a good thing because it's saturated fat and is considered by doctors as a major contributor to high cholesterol and coronary artery disease — one of the top killers of Americans. Drink a glass of whole milk and you just downed the equivalent of two teaspoons of grease, half of which is the bad fat. Is cheese okay? Nope, a slice is concentrated butterfat.

If you are over three years old we strongly encourage you not to go near whole milk since it doesn't contain anything you need as a punching and kicking martial artist.

One and Two Percent Milk

While many two percent milk cartons read "low fat," the truth is that the number refers to the percentage of the milk's weight that is fat. So when talking calories, two percent means that 45 percent of the total calories come from fat. This isn't good. One percent milk is better, but just a little. Choose skim milk, which has no fat at all.

Skim Milk: The Good

If you can tolerate milk, drink only skim as it completely eliminates from the equation that heart-hating and flab-producing butterfat. Equally as important is that skim milk actually contains more calcium than whole milk, so critically important for maintaining strong bones. As a martial artist, you want steel in those bones of yours since you bang against opponents when sparring and bounce off the floor when grappling. Adults can get up to 75 percent of their daily calcium requirement when drinking two or three glasses of skim each day.

Skim milk is also a good way to control your weight. A glass with your meal helps you to feel full so you eat a smaller portion of mashed potatoes. The same is true with whole milk, but you get fewer calories with skim. If you are a whole milk drinker, here is an easy way to drop 10 pounds by this same date next year. Instead of putting that butterfat-rich whole milk on your bran flakes in the morning, use skim milk. Just that small change will trim 10 pounds from your figure in only 12 months.

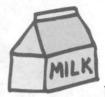

Milk Facts

- Don't drink it at all if you are lactose intolerant

- There are dairy products, including milk, for people with lactose intolerance

- Whole milk bad, skim milk good

- Whole milk is loaded with killer butterfat

- Two percent means that 45 percent of the calories comes from fat

- Skim milk has less calories and more calcium than whole milk

- Skim milk makes you feel full, so that you eat less

- One glass of skim provides eight grams of protein

Fast Facts

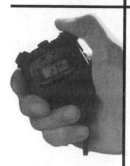

- Your foundation-eating plan is based on your regular training regimen and used on routine days. Once established, you can tweak it depending on the specifics of your daily training.

- If you aren't eating with someone or cooking for or with someone, it can be hard to stay on course to eat nutritiously. If this is you, well, snap out of it and stop being so helpless.

- After a hard martial arts workout or a grueling all-day competition, too many fighters "refuel" with junk so that their exhausted, depleted bodies have to struggle to find what few, lonely nutrients there are, and then send them out to try to repair the wear and tear from all the kicking and punching.

- If you walk into a fast food joint armed with the same incredible discipline you have developed in your martial arts training, there are actually a few healthy things you can eat.

- Enter a fast food restaurant telling yourself that you are going to eat just enough to eliminate your hunger for a couple of hours until you can eat something more nutritious.

- Movie snack bar candy is usually industrial sized, so you might want to bring a smaller one from home and sneak it in, or better yet, sneak in a health bar.

- Dirt Day is one day a week when you get to have a meal of anything you want: hamburgers, ice cream, pizza, whatever. Think of it as a reward for your other six days of disciplined eating.

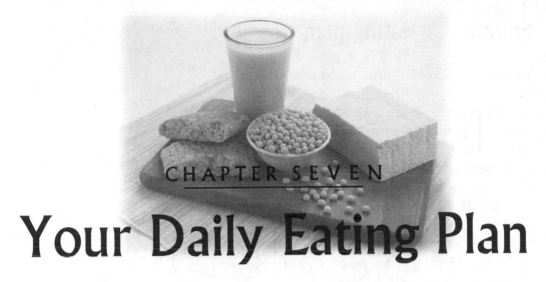

CHAPTER SEVEN

Your Daily Eating Plan

It would take a monster-sized volume to include all the meals applicable to the many needs of martial artists. There would need to be menus for fighters wanting to lose weight, gain weight and maintain their weight; menus for fighters preparing for competition and a grueling belt exam; meals for weight lifting days, aerobics days and rest days; and meals for fast weight loss plans and for all-day seminars. Such an array of menu plans would necessitate dozens of pages, wasted pages since few people would use them, anyway.

If you are interested in collecting and following recipes, know that there are dozens of magazines and cookbooks on the market that offer healthy meals to fit your needs. Most include carb, protein and fat grams, and the total calories of the meal. But if you have no intentions of ever reading a cookbook, you still have to make an effort to know the contents of what you whip up. Happily, it's not much of an effort since there are

little booklets available near the checkout counters at most grocery stores and in bookstores that provide basic information as to the nutritional content in common foods. Some even list fast-food items.

Whether you are a white belt or a black belt in the kitchen, it's important that you first establish a foundation, a base for your carb, protein and fat needs. Once you have that in place, you can easily modify it depending on your needs.

Foundation-eating plan

Your foundation-eating plan is based on your regular training regimen and used on routine days. See Chapter 3 to determine your daily protein, carb and fat needs and how to slice the pie. Here are three suggestions:

• If you lift weights four or five days a week and train in the martial arts two days a week, your foundation-diet should consist of a high percentage of protein.

• If you train four or five days a week in the martial arts and lift weights only two days a week, your founda-tion-diet should emphasize quality carbs.

• If you jog three miles a day, five days a week and train in the martial arts on your two off days, your foundation-diet should be even higher in quality carbs.

Once you have established a foundation-eating plan, you are in a position to tweak it depending on the specifics of your daily training. Here are some ideas:

• If you lift weights four or five days a week and your diet emphasizes protein, reduce the protein on your martial arts days and take a bigger slice of carbs.

• If you normally practice your martial arts five days a week, eating a large slice of carbs each day, eat fewer on your two lifting days and increase your protein slice.

• If you are a five-days-a-week jogger, reduce your carbs a little on your martial arts days.

As always, you need to experiment to see what works best for your particular body and lifestyle.

Let's see how two good looking, suave and debonair guys who train in the martial arts and lift weights manage their foundation-eating plan. Of course we are talking about us. The purpose is to show you how average, but hard-training fighters follow disciplined eating plans that are surprising normal. We don't mix strange concoctions or drink blood from stray dogs. Our meals are simple and basic. If there is anything unique about our approach it's that we both have good discipline to stay on course. Most of the time.

How Christensen Does It

Christensen has always been cursed with a slow metabolism and it's gotten slower every time he has a birthday. As a full-time writer, his work is mostly sedentary, though he tries to work out every day. He lifts weights three times a week and trains in the martial arts three or four days a week; at least two of the martial arts sessions are intense. His weight training sessions are light because they are aimed at increasing power in his martial arts movements, as opposed to lifting to gain additional size. In fact, he deliberately trains not to increase muscles mass.

Christensen's foundation eating plan is to take in six small meals a day, spaced about three hours apart, eating 10 to 20 percent fat, 30 percent protein and 50 to 60 percent carbs. On those days he only lifts weights, he increases the protein to 40 percent, robbing 10 percent from the carb side.

His breakfasts are always the same: An English muffin with an olive oil spread, at least two tablespoons of peanut butter and a piece of fruit, totaling around 500 calories. At midmorning, he has an apple and a protein drink for about 250 calories, and for lunch, he has three ounces of lean meat and a vegetable for about 400 calories. At mid-afternoon it's another piece of fruit and a small bag of peanuts for about 250 calories. For dinner, it's meat again and a vegetable for 400 calories. A mid-evening snack usually consists of a fat-free yogurt with fruit for 150 calories. All this adds up to about 1,950 calories. Counting his fat-free coffee cream, a snuck spoonful of peanut butter or a small chunk of chocolate, Christensen ends the day at around 2,150 calories, a plan he follows about five days a week. On the other two days he follows the plan until dinner, and then he dines out where he inevitably takes in quite a few more calories than usual.

When he wants to drop a few pounds, he increases his cardio training, using the martial arts, and cuts back on one or both days of the high-calorie evening meals. He still goes out, but he chooses carefully what he eats and pays close attention to the calorie count. If the restaurant offers large servings, he eats only half. No desert and no beer.

Since he normally follows a healthy diet and training regimen, all he has to do differently to drop two or three pounds is increase his cardio training a little and be calorie conscious at least six days a week, or all seven if he needs it off in a hurry. He never goes hungry, he maintains an even energy level, and is never far off peak condition.

How Demeere Does It

Co-author Demeere is fortunate in that he has a relatively fast metabolism. The downside is that he gets hungry faster than most people, so eating frequent meals is critical to keep his stomach gnawing at bay and to maintain an even energy level throughout the day. If for whatever reason he can't eat every three hours, he turns into a famished, salivating beast, tearing and ripping into his next meal with snarls, growls and threatening glares at anyone who comes near. Eating like this usually leads to devouring too many calories and ultimately to unwanted weight gain. This is why he makes every effort to stay on schedule.

As a personal trainer, Demeere must consider two dietary factors during his day. First, since it can be a real challenge to eat healthily when on the road between clients, he often brown bags nutritious sandwiches from home, or if he eats out, he knows where all the quality eateries are. Second, although teaching martial arts is usually not as demanding as is his personal training, it's nonetheless vigorous physical activity. As such, he factors in additional calories to get him through his teaching schedule, as well as his own training.

Demeere's personal daily training regimen consists of one to two hours of martial arts each day, and intensive aerobic and weight training five days a week. He fuels this tremendous output with a nutritional strategy of 50- to 60-percent carbs, 30- to 35-percent protein and the rest fat.

Breakfast is usually several slices of bread with low-fat cheese, tuna or chicken, sometimes low-fat fruit yogurt, and coffee. This adds up to between 650 and 800 calories, 60 percent of which are carbs to give him enough energy to get through his training a couple of hours after breakfast. On off days or when he doesn't train immediately after breakfast, he eats only two or three slices of bread, or muesli, a healthy cereal with fat-free milk, to keep the calories between 400 and 500.

Once he finishes working out at the gym around lunchtime, he consumes a protein shake of around 300 calories to help repair the muscle tissue. If he has clients after lunch, he eats around 450 calories worth of fruit and sandwiches made of a low-fat spread. If he doesn't have to work, he limits his intake to about 300 to 350 calories.

Early in the afternoon, he usually has a few pieces of fruit or a carbohydrate-rich energy bar to keep his blood sugar level steady. Dinner is a hot meal comprised mainly of lean meat (poultry, fish or beef) and carbohydrates (pasta, brown rice or potatoes) and vegetables for fiber. Ever aware of the predominance of fat in our Western diets, he grills and steams instead of baking. He uses a wok to cook vegetables and meat, and sprinkles it with unsaturated oil instead of margarine or butter. Since dinner usually precedes more martial arts training, he takes in at least 600 calories, sometimes more. After his evening class and before he crashes into bed, he has a little yogurt with fruit.

In the end, his basic nutritional plan weighs in somewhere around 2300 and 2500 calories. But it's not always easy since he is a hardcore chocolate-addict. Living in Belgium is a true test of his discipline, as he is exposed almost daily to the absolute best in goodies for the sweet tooth. If Demeere weren't disciplined, he would devour pounds of it every day, so that in no time he would have to be rolled out onto the training floor. To avoid going stark raving mad, he allows himself either a little chocolate during breakfast or as a snack on his "Dirt Day" (discussed later in this chapter).

Being human and all, there are those times when his bathroom scales mocks him by pointing at numbers higher than he likes, almost always the result of overindulging in chocolate. When that happens, he turns up the discipline to cut back on the evil stuff and trains a little harder to shed the extra pounds.

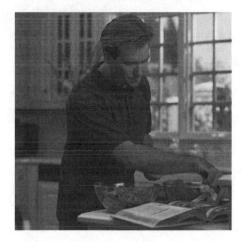

For Bachelors and Bachelorettes

It's not that single martial artists are helpless in the kitchen (though some are), it's more an issue of motivation. If you aren't eating with someone or cooking for or with someone, it can be hard to stay on course to eat nutritiously. If this is you, well, snap out of it and stop being so helpless. If you are organized enough to get up in the morning and trudge off to work or school, and later go to your martial arts class, you can certainly plan a simple, healthy way of eating. Your work, school and especially your training require that you are healthy and energetic, qualities derived from good nutrition. The problem is that too many people put more effort into their fashion statement than into selecting the right fuel for their bodies.

Two Breakfast Ideas

• Don't buy breakfast cereal based on the free toy inside, but choose one loaded with nutrients and low on fat and sugar. Pick up half a gallon of skim milk and a container of whey protein. Instead of putting sugar on your cereal, sprinkle on a couple of t-spoons of vanilla protein. Add a fruit of your liking and you got yourself a 500-calorie breakfast to kick start your day.

• On Sunday, scramble six eggs in a little olive oil with low-fat cheese, some lean ham, chicken or turkey, and onion. Pour the ingredients equally into three burrito shells, add as much no-calorie taco sauce as you want and roll them up. Wrap them in plastic wrap and toss them into the refrigerator or freezer. On Monday morning, nuke one for 40 seconds and munch on it as you dress. Eat a pear or banana and you got yourself about 500 nutrient-packed calories to head out into the world.

Two Mid-morning Snack Ideas

• Find a nutrition bar you like. Yes, many of them taste like yesterday's dog food, but if you look long enough you can find one that you will look forward too all morning. Make sure it's nutrition rich, with at least 15 grams of protein and doesn't exceed 300 calories. Eat it slowly so you enjoy every bite and it satisfies your hunger for a sweet snack.

- Toss your favorite fruit and a small carton of skim milk into your lunch bag. The fruit provides some quality carbs and the milk supplies your bod' with eight grams of protein, all for about 200 calories.

Two Lunch Ideas

- If you had cereal for breakfast, take your burrito for lunch, and include some carrot and celery sticks. Granted, this isn't too exciting, but it keeps your energy level even and supplies your body with 400 quality calories.

- Load your lunch bag with a low-fat yogurt cup, a couple of fig bars and a carton of skim milk. This gives you 400 calories and 16 grams of protein

Two Mid-afternoon Ideas

- To help get through the afternoon slump and satisfy your sweet tooth, enjoy a cup of coffee as you munch slowly on a chocolate, peanut butter or fruit granola bar. All this for only 120 calories.

- Have a pre-mixed protein drink (store bought or one you mixed at home and brought with you). It's nutrient rich, contains around 20 grams of protein at 150 calories when mixed with water.

Two Dinner Ideas

- Your martial arts class is at 7 PM, so at 5 PM eat a plate of spaghetti with low-cal sauce and a cup of veggies. This supplies about 500 calories, most of which are carbs to fuel your kicks and punches for a couple of hours.

- Have a sandwich. A couple slices of vitamin fortified whole-wheat bread, a slice of cheese, lettuce, tomatoes and half an avocado. Wash it down with a cup of milk. This gives you lots of carbs and 500 calories of energy for your training.

Two Mid-evening Snacks

- If your class involved lots of strength-building drills, such as horse-stance squats and push-ups, have a protein drink as soon after training as possible. This gives you around 20 grams to repair and build your tired muscles, at about 150 calories.

- If your class was primarily cardio, such as high-rep punching, kicking drills and lots of sparring, you need to replenish your energy reserves with quality carbs. Eat 200 hundred calories of leftover spaghetti or a couple pieces of fruit.

The above suggestions supply a body with 2000 calories a day. If you are trying to lose weight by taking in only 1,800 a day (which is dangerously close to being unhealthy), simply cut 75 calories from each of your major meals. If you have determined you should eat 3,000 a day, you are in hog heaven. Pump up the calories in all your meals, but just make sure they are quality ones.

If all this seems like a lot of work and preplanning, it just might be at first, but soon it becomes part of your day. You already plan what you are going to wear, your route to work or school, how your day will unfold, your route to your martial arts class, and even what you are going to focus on in your training. How much harder is it to plan what you are going to eat? All things considered, determining your fueling needs is arguably the most important thing you do for yourself each day.

You Can Eat Healthily at Fast Food Joints

Let's say you own a high-performance racecar propelled by a state-of-the art, technologically superior engine. To run at its absolute optimum, it needs jet fuel designed by the most brilliant minds at NASA. Today you plan to race your car, but instead of filling it with that high-tech jet fuel, you dump a couple scoops of sugar in the tank, a whole lot of hamburger grease, a handful of salt and a 64-ounce cup of soda pop.

Of course, no one would do this to their personal car, though a vandal would to criminally destroy the inner mechanisms of the machine. Sadly, millions or people criminally vandalize

their own bodies daily by dumping toxic substances into their systems — including hard training martial artists. As instructors, we have seen students walk into to class munching on the last greasy bite of a burger and fries bought at a drive-up. These people are vandals, deliberately trashing the inner mechanisms of their high-performance bodies. There is no way they can perform at their optimum with this garbage in their hardworking bloodstreams, muscles, joints, cartilage, lungs, brains, and all the little but nonetheless vital parts used in the martial arts.

Their typical argument is this: "Hey, I get off work just before class and I always grab a burger and a shake on the way. And I do fine. I'm moving up the belt ranks and I win lots of trophies."

Fine, but the questions that must be asked are: How much better could they do if they fed their bodies quality food instead of grease and sugar? How many fewer injuries would they have if they had quality nutrients racing to their tired body parts instead of all that fat and salt? How much more energy would they have if they ate two hours before training? How much faster would they recuperate from their hard workouts? How much stronger would they be? Faster? More flexible?

After a hard martial arts workout or a grueling all-day competition, too many fighters opt for fast food on their way home. Their bodies are tired and begging for high quality protein, carbs, vitamins and minerals to replenish all that was lost, but they yield to what is convenient and what satisfies their desire for sugar-rich, high-fat food. They "refuel" with junk so that their exhausted, depleted bodies have to struggle to find what few, lonely nutrients there are, and then send them out to try to repair the wear and tear from all the kicking and punching. Will there be enough to completely replenish the exhausted bodies before they have to train again? Probably not. Will it take a toll if this becomes a repeated cycle? You betcha. Some people last longer than others, and there is that one out of a thousand who gets away with it forever, but most suffer with ill health, weakened muscles and chronic injuries.

Calories, Lots of Them

Studies show that the average fast-food meal yields 1,200 to 1,700 calories, all of which are usually high in fat, cholesterol and sodium (salt). Keep in mind that calories can double when deep-fried, and that innocent looking swipe of special sauce across a hamburger bun can add at least 100 more. That milkshake that looks so good in the poster behind the counter adds 500 to 1000 calories to your butt, the same number you burn when you jog for 60 minutes. Two or three shakes a week and you won't be able to lift your thunder thighs to throw one of your fancy kicks. Surely, hotcakes from the drive-thru are okay, right? Sorry, but they contain a big 600 calories (if you are conservative with the butter

and syrup) designed to turn you into the karate-class slug.

Here are some other menu items that might seem inconsequential but, along with the triple burgers and fries served in a bag the size of a backpack, do nothing for your health and progress in the martial arts:

• Sauces of all kinds (high fat and calories)

• Chicken nuggets (grease, skin and very little meat)

• Cheese sauce (gooey fat to clog your arteries)

• Fish sandwich (grease)

• Croissants (lots of fat)

• Anything fried: burger, fish, chicken (grease, grease, grease)

• Fries (extreme grease and sodium)

• Onion rings (extreme grease and sodium)

• Salad dressing (extremely high in fat and calories)

Encourage your opponent to eat this junk, but you want to duck it like a spinning backfist.

Let's examine a few popular fast foods. The columns on the left reveal what the "food" contains, and the column on the right shows what the average fighter should get each day. Remember, these represent just one meal. Are any of your favorite fast foods listed here?

Burger: Quarter-Pound Cheeseburger, large fries, 16 oz. soda (McDonald's®)

Meal	Recommended daily intake
1,166 calories	2,000-2,700 calories
51 g fat	No more than 50-80 g
95 mg cholesterol	No more than 300 mg
1,450 mg sodium	No more than 1,100-3,300 mg

Pizza: Four slices of sausage and mushroom pizza, 16 oz. soda (Domino's®)

Meal	Recommended daily intake
1,000 calories	2,000-2,700 calories
28 g fat	No more than 50-80 g
62 mg cholesterol	No more than 300 mg
2,302 mg sodium	No more than 1,100-3,300 mg

Chicken: Two pieces of fried chicken (breast and wing), buttermilk biscuit, mashed potatoes and gravy, corn-on-the-cob, 16 oz. soda (KFC®)

Meal	Recommended daily intake
1,232 calories	2,000-2,700 calories
57 g fat	No more than 50-80 g
157 mg cholesterol	No more than 300 mg
2,276 mg sodium	No more than 1,100-3,300 mg

Taco: Taco salad, 16 oz. soda (Taco Bell®)

Meal	Recommended daily intake
1,057 calories	2,000-2,700 calories
55 g fat	No more than 50-80 g
80 mg cholesterol	No more than 300 mg
1,620 mg sodium	No more than 1,100-3,300 mg

It Takes Discipline and Knowledge to Eat Right at the Drive-up

If you walk into a fast food joint armed with the same incredible discipline you have developed in your martial arts training, there are actually a few healthy things you can eat. The underscored word here is discipline. If you lack it, or what little you have is fragile and crumbles easily under temptation, there is nothing good about fast food joints for you. It's especially important to avoid eating breakfast in them, since you are usually hungry in the morning and in need of good nutrients to help you start the day. Their bright colors, delicious smells and many images of foods that tempt and tease your senses, it's oh-so-easy to gorge yourself on pancakes, sausages and other fat-, sugar-, and cholesterol-dense foods.

Eat just enough to get by   While a fast food joint might be your only option, consider it your only option right now. Enter the place telling yourself that you are going to eat just enough to eliminate your hunger for a couple of hours until you can eat something more nutritious. As always, eat slowly to give your brain time to get the message that your stomach is full. This is especially important when you are in a place where it's so easy to order one more burger or one more bag of fries. It's all about disciplined and strategic thinking so that you can resist all the goodies these places offer.

Name familiarity   Say you are on the highway traveling to a tournament and the only food available are fast food joints at every exit. Not the best situation, but the good news is that you know what type of food these familiar places offer. Consider the following:

- The big name eateries have basically the same menus across the country. This is helpful when you know that a burger joint offers a filling, 350-calorie veggie burger, or a baked potato without all that heart-clogging sour cream.

- Avoid the mega-huge meals and order regular size or child's size. Be cautious with the sodas, too, as some are served in cups large enough to have their own tides, not to mention voluminous calories, caffeine and sugar. Instead, ask for ice water, ice tea or diet soda. Nutritionally, your best bet is always skim milk.

- Some fast food joints post the nutritional content of their offerings on a wall, or you can ask to see a list. If they don't have one, pull out your trusty little calorie counter booklet.

Healthy choices   Here are some fast-food menu items that are low in fat, sugar and calories, while containing healthy nutrients:

- Grilled chicken sandwiches with tomatoes and onions.

- Roasted or broiled chicken. Always remove the skin from any chicken item to reduce the fat content even more.

- Baked potato without all the fixings.

- Fat-free milk.

- Salad with the dressing on the side, preferable fat-free. If you are very hungry, order an extra salad instead of an extra burger. The raw vegetables fill you and reduce the risk of overeating.

- Single burger (regular or kid-size) with tomatoes and onions.

- Burger, but eat it with only one bun (this can be a little messy)

- Burger, but eat only the goodies inside, not the buns.

Check out the internet sites below to learn more about calories and fat grams of menu items in all the mainstream fast food places. Don't get depressed because your favorites are outrageously high in everything that is bad for your health and your progress in the martial arts. Think positively and strategically. First, memorize the ingredients of your favorite fast food items so you know what you are getting on your Dirt Day or those rare occasions when you decide to reward yourself with a special treat. Also memorize those few items on the menu that are relatively nutritious, filling and low in calories, fat, sugar, and salt.

You can eat at fast food joints, but you need to do so with discipline and knowledge. Ever heard those two words mentioned in your martial arts training?

Calorie Counters: Fast food nutritional guide:

http://www.calorie-counters.net

Fast food facts:

http://www.kenkuhl.com/fastfood

At the Movies

Use your discipline at the movies, too. Know that it's easy to get caught up in a film and "zone out" as you mindlessly shovel in the junk. If you have to eat popcorn, and it's not a bad thing as long as it's not floating in butter and coated in salt, order the child's box and share it with your date (or give the last half to that weird guy with the overcoat talking to himself a couple of seats down). Snackbar candy is usually industrial sized, so you might want to bring a smaller one from home and sneak it in, or better yet, sneak in a health bar (if you get caught, don't drag us into your court case).

Check out these charts to see how you can eat relatively healthy.

Burger: Hamburger, small fries, 16 oz. soda (McDonald's)

Meal	Recommended daily intake
481 calories	2,000-2,700 calories
19 g fat	No more than 50-80 g
30 mg cholesterol	No more than 300 mg
665 mg sodium	No more than 1,100-3,300 mg

Pizza: Three slices of cheese pizza, 16 oz. diet soda (Domino's)

Meal	Recommended daily intake
516 calories	2,000-2,700 calories
15 g fat	No more than 50-80 g
29 mg cholesterol	No more than 300 mg
1,470 mg sodium	No more than 1,100-3,300 mg

Chicken: One piece of fried chicken (wing), mashed potatoes and gravy, coleslaw, 16 oz. diet soda (KFC)

Meal	Recommended daily intake
373 calories	2,000-2,700 calories
19 g fat	No more than 50-80 g
46 mg cholesterol	No more than 300 mg
943 mg sodium	No more than 1,100-3,300 mg

Taco: Three light tacos, 16 oz. diet soda (Taco Bell)

Meal	Recommended daily intake
420 calories	2,000-2,700 calories
15 g fat	No more than 50-80 g
60 mg cholesterol	No more than 300 mg
840 mg sodium	No more than 1,100-3,300 mg

Dirt Day

No, this isn't about eating dirt, though no doubt there is someone, somewhere (California comes to mind) thinking up a way to charge desperate people for little cartons of magic dirt from a mountain in Central America that "melts away the pounds." We wish, but in this case the term refers to one glorious day a week when you can eat anything you want.

Say you have been watching the fat intake and counting calories for six days in a row. Your discipline has been ironclad and you can hold your head high with pride for a job well done. Your reward is that on the seventh day you can have a big piece of your favorite cake and a scoop of ice cream. Or a pizza and a drink. Or a burger and a shake. Get the idea? Garbage food. Junk food. Dirt.

The concept is simple: Dirt Day provides you with a happy goal as you follow your strict regimen throughout the week. If your Dirt Day is a Saturday, and on Thursday you find that your discipline is beginning to wane, a mental image of Dirt Day — I get french fries and greasy chicken in just two more days — strengthens your will to stay on course. Think of it as a dangling carrot; a tasty goal; the light at the end of the tunnel; something to look forward to when hunger, cravings and temptation taunts your will.

Martial arts champion and movie action star Marc Dacascos follows a diet of good protein and vegetables throughout the week, but on weekends, he relaxes his regimen. He says: "Weekends, that's my playtime so I eat whatever I want. Occasionally a glass of red wine; I just can't take very much of it." [24]

Maybe you possess discipline of steel and don't need a weekly Dirt Day. Consider having one every two weeks or, do as one top athlete said on a television talk show: "I take one day a month and eat whatever I want."

Kick boxer and author Martina Sprague says she eats a burger and fries only twice a year. Through trial and error you discover what works best for you.

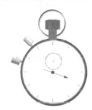

It's Really Not All Day

Dirt Day is actually a misnomer because it isn't a good idea to eat poorly all day long, since it's frighteningly easy to undo everything you have struggled for over the last six days. It's better to just have a dirt meal, or a dirt treat because as you know by now, calories add up at a cursedly fast rate. A breakfast of hotcakes and sausage, a triple burger and milkshake for lunch and a big evening meal can easily contain more calories than you cut the previous six days.

Savor the Moment

When Dirt Day finally rolls around, don't attack your treat like a starving, mad dog tearing into fresh road kill. You have waited six days for this or longer, so take your time and s-a-v-o-r what you have been craving. Pick up a morsel on the end of your fork, smell it, taste it, nibble it, and then chew it slowly and thoroughly, delighting in the flavors you have been missing.

By making a long, wonderful moment out of the eating experience, you completely satisfy your tastebuds and enjoy a more fulfilling treat. As discussed previously, when you gorge food you are more apt to overeat because you eat faster than your brain can register that you are full. Eat slowly and savor each bite so that you know when you are satisfied and therefore better able to resist a second helping.

Not for Everyone

There are those who say that a Dirt Day is a bad idea, and we agree there are some good arguments against it. Perhaps the biggest one is that some people are wired in such a way that a Dirt Day would be harmful to them. For example, there are people who, once they make the decision to eat healthily, stick to their decision religiously, looking away even when the most sinfully delicious restaurant desert tray is presented. But should they purposely include a Dirt Day into their regimen, they lose their will and switch to eating junk food with the same fervor they had when eating only healthily. One treat leads to a second and then to a third, and before they can say "More whipping cream, please," they have destroyed the progress made in previous days and are packing on additional pounds. It's possible that this mental quirk is a symptom of an eating disorder, in which case it's important to seek guidance from a doctor.

Dirt Day Variations

You may discover, as co-author Christensen did during his hardcore bodybuilding days, a Dirt Day was not worth how he felt afterwards. His often consisted of a triple scoop of ice cream hidden under a thick coating of chocolate fudge. He says that though he enjoyed the heck out of it, it left him hyped and buzzing like a moth around a light bulb. If he ate it in the evening, he was so buzzed that he couldn't sleep. No doubt Christensen reacted strongly to the treat because during the previous week he ate no sugar at all and very little fat. He eventually disciplined himself to one scoop of ice cream or had other treats that weren't so sugar intense.

How about a little bit of dirt every day? (Okay, now we're talkin'!) This works only if you have great discipline. If you are one of those people who can't stop with one little treat, dirt every day isn't for you. But if you can control it and want to have a treat every day, remember this: Whether you are trying to lose weight or maintain, it's all about calories, so you got to count them. You have to factor in the daily treat.

Use your discipline Christensen likes cookies and has the occasional one at lunch after he has eaten meat and veggies. An average sized cookie has 100 or more calories, the meat and veggies about 300, which adds up to a 400-calorie lunch, the exact amount he wants. While the cookie satisfies his sweet tooth, it's not filling. So on those noondays when he is really hungry, he eats an extra 100 calories of food that better satiates his hunger, such as tuna, chicken and veggies. Since they don't satisfy his sweet tooth but his calorie quota has been met, he draws on his discipline to skip the sweet treat.

Amazon.com's Special Interests editor, Jenny Brown, interviewed Tae-Bo master Billy Blanks in Seattle after a demonstration. When asked about his diet, Blanks said, "I like Pepsi cola. Once in a while I'll eat a cheeseburger, but I don't eat and drink this all the time. But when I'm getting ready for something and I need to be in the best shape that I can be in, then I'll cut out drinking the soda." [25]

Full-contact champion Frank Shamrock believes that from a psychological standpoint it's important to have a little dirt. "I eat junk," he says. "Burgers, pizza, stuff like that. Your body can handle it; just don't overdo it. If you eat healthy stuff, lean protein, vegetables, fruits, stuff like that, you can have two 'cheat' days a week to keep you honest.

If you pig out two days a week, then it's not like you're bound to this restricted diet your whole life." [26] While two Dirt days works for the very hard training, calorie-burning Shamrock, we advise one day.

Dirt Day as a Motivator

Dirt Day may be the only thing that keeps you motivated, but be careful not to allow your anticipation of it to dominate your every thought. In the beginning of a new lifestyle-eating plan, many people find it so excruciatingly difficult to stay away from high-sugar, high-carb and high-fat foods that they spend virtually every waking moment dreaming of the perceived joys of chocolate and french fries. As mentioned earlier, obsessing about food makes you vulnerable to binging and overeating. Strive to control your thoughts. When an ice cream sundae pops into your mind, throw backfists, 3 sets of 10 reps. When a burger and fries call your name, do 4 sets of 10 reps of whatever kick needs extra work.

How to Transition

Dirt Day can be used as a transition to help develop sound nutritional habits. Maybe a double Dirt Day per week would work in the beginning, such as Wednesdays and Saturdays (do we have good ideas, or what?). On those two days, you are allowed one piece of junk, as a main course (fries and burgers) or as a desert treat (butterscotch pudding or cookie dough ice cream) following your usual healthy meal. This way, you get to chow down on a goodie every three days.

To implement this plan, circle the days on your calendar at the beginning of the month. For two weeks you get two Dirt Days a week. Beginning the third week, you add an extra day between each Dirt Day and continue to add a day every week over the course of the next two or three weeks until you are enjoying just one Dirt Day a week. When you arrive at this stage, feel good about yourself and your accomplishment, but don't celebrate with cake (we read your mind didn't we?). Instead, buy yourself an inedible present, like a T-shirt.

Whether you have Dirt Day twice a week, once a week, every two weeks, once a month, or a little one every day, the crucial element that makes it work is knowledge of yourself, knowledge of calories and discipline. Dirt Day is a way to reward yourself for your efforts and keep your discipline strong. As always, however, you need to proceed wisely and with a goal of being fighting fit in the forefront of your mind.

Fast Facts

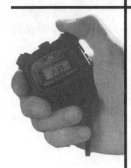

- By itself, repping out crunches until your belly button pops off like a wine cork won't trim your waistline.

- Hard bag work trims the abs more than crunches because it burns more calories.

- While having a gut can cause back problems, slow your mobility and make your heart work extra hard, it doesn't necessarily make you obese.

- High Intensity Interval Training, HIIT, gets its fuel primarily from carbs and to a lesser degree from fat, but due to its high intensity, the total number of calories burned is much higher than when doing low intensity training.

- Here is what this means for your love handles. HIIT burns your body fat up to 50 percent more efficiently than jogging around potholes or pedaling to nowhere.

- People who split their aerobic activity — say half in the morning and half in the evening — burn more fat than people who do it all at once.

- Park 10 minutes from work or school and walk as fast as you can to it, and in the afternoon walk back to your car as fast as you can. That is 20 minutes of light aerobics. That night in class, do your regular workout and then hit the heavy bag for 20 minutes after class, for a grand total of 40 minutes of cardio for the day.

- When you first get up in the morning and you haven't eaten carbohydrates for several hours, your body gets energy from your fat, but only if you train aerobically, which means at moderate to low intensity.

- Since the abs are so instrumental in delivering explosive, pile driving leg attacks, you can use your kicks to develop your midsection.

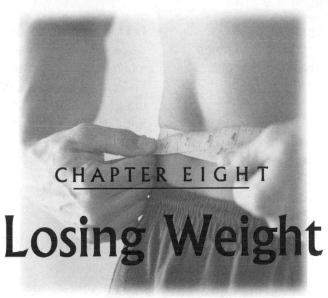

CHAPTER EIGHT

Losing Weight

How to Use Martial Arts to Get Rid of Your Gut

Bruce Lee, Joe Lewis, Bill Wallace and Jean-Claude Van Damme are four of the most famous faces in the United States martial arts scene and, as such, thousands of students have tried to copy not only their fighting techniques, but their physical appearance as well, especially their rock hard abdominals. Let's explore how you can achieve similar results through diet and exercise, whether your physique is wiry, like Lee's was, bulky, like Lewis's and Van Damme's, or lean and athletic like Wallace's.

Have Realistic Expectations

Not everyone is blessed with the genetics to have a well-defined physique all year long. In the world of athletics, there are hard gainers and easy gainers. While many of the models on the covers of fitness and martial arts magazines are easy gainers and always look that way, there are a few not so blessed who must work hard and sweat blood for that awesome appearance they maintain for only a few days on each side of their photo shoots. Know that just because you were not in line when the exceptional genes were handed out, doesn't mean you can't achieve a strong, or even ripped midsection. (As mentioned before, you don't have to have defined abdominals to do well in the martial arts).

Approach Your Objective from Different Angles

By itself, repping out crunches until your belly button pops off like a wine cork won't trim your waistline, nor will hitting the bag for an hour every day. Actually, doing hard bag work to develop power, form and aerobic conditioning does more to trim the tummy than crunches because it burns more calories. But to get the best results

— muscle development and reduced fat — you need to take an integrated approach by incorporating aerobic training, proper eating, free-hand exercises and weight training.

Note: While we discuss aerobics and various eating plans throughout this book, weight training is discussed only briefly, mostly in Chapter 11 where we provide basic exercises to build power and burn calories. The subject of weight training is an incredibly vast one far beyond this book's scope. We encourage you, however, to learn all you can about it and incorporate it into your training regimen. Co-author Christensen's book *Fighting Power: How to Develop Explosive Punches, Kicks, Blocks and Grappling* contains lots of strength developing workouts for martial artists. It's available on his site www.lwcbooks.com (yes, that was a shameless plug).

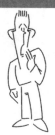

Gut Facts

While having a gut can cause back problems, slow your mobility and make your heart work extra hard, it doesn't necessarily make you obese. Some people stock most of their fat around their waist but carry only a little on the rest of their body. There are even those with protruding stomachs who actually have a lower body fat percentage than those who appear mildly overweight.

Let's examine various forms of aerobics using your fighting art and then look at a few hard but highly effective abdominal exercises. When you integrate these into your training along with good nutrition habits, you will be on a fast track to a lean and powerful mid-section.

Negative Caloric Balance

In the world of calories, there are those you eat and those you burn. If on a given day you don't change your physical activities but you reduce the number of calories you consume, you end your day with a negative caloric balance. For example, say you need 3,000 calories to maintain your weight but today you take in only 2,700. This means that at the end of the day you lost a little weight, though not much and no one will notice. If you were a bookkeeper, you would place your daily calories in the red column to denote a loss. Now, if instead of reducing the calories you eat, you take in the same 3,000 but train hard to burn 300 extra, you again end your day with 2,700 and your calorie count in the red column. So in a nutshell, you lose a little weight when you cut 300 calories out of your diet and you lose a little weight when you eat the same as usual but burn an extra 300 in training.

Are you ahead of us here and see where this going? You are right if you figured that by cutting back 300 calories from your chow and burning an extra 300 through your training, you end the day with 600 calories in the red column. This means that should you continue to double up, so to speak, your gut will shrink twice as fast than if you just used one approach to delete 300 calories a day. Admittedly, using both methods is a tough way to get a calorie deficit, one that takes a lot of willpower, but so what? You are a martial artist and you laugh in the face of tough.

Caution: It was mentioned earlier that your body doesn't like radical changes. While a total of 600 calories in the red is doable, it's unwise and dangerous to take the more-is-better approach and cut, say, 800 calories from your diet and then burn another 650 by sparring until you collapse. That is a fast path to overexertion, overtraining, injury, and depleting your nutritional reserves.

Negative caloric balance is an effective way to lose your belly, but only if you approach the task progressively and conservatively. Obviously, you don't want a flat stomach but then have a knee in traction because you drastically cut calories and vital nutrition, overtrained and over strained.

Experiment with any of the many eating plans in this book to reduce your daily intake by 300 calories. Once you find one that fits you like a glove — meaning you can follow it with little or no sense of depriving yourself — choose one or more of the following aerobic activities that you like to burn another 300 calories.

High Intensity Interval Training (HIIT)

Co-author Christensen touched on this training concept in his book *Fighter's Fact Book*, but because it's such an effective fat burning device it's worth elaborating on here. High intensity interval training (HIIT) has been around since the late 1980s, although *Muscle Media* magazine and writer Shawn Phillips brought it into prominence in the late 1990s. It's a tough training regimen that when combined with a minor reduction in calories, the 300 per day we just discussed, strips off the el lard-o from your el frame-o in a short time-o. Though it was initially designed for the barbell crowd, we found it works wonders for martial artists, too.

How it Works

Have you ever noticed those people in health clubs pedaling away on stationary bicycles with their heads buried in the most recent Danielle Steele novel? Notice how they all wear "uniforms:" baggy sweats pants with either a baggy sweatshirt or an untucked, oversized T-shirt. They wear these because they are overweight and trying to hide the fact, though no one is fooled. They look rather like hamsters in a cage, pedaling madly to nowhere, bored and getting little or no results for their efforts. Bless their hearts because they probably don't want to pedal for 60 minutes at a shot, but they do so in hopes that in time they can get out of those uniforms and into tank tops and shorts.

They also pump mindlessly and uselessly because health club trainers tell them to. Most trainers know that HIIT is a more effective way to burn fat, but they also know that it would be a risk to have new, overweight club members do it (it's bad for business to have dead members lying about on the floor). Besides the physical stress on the untrained and out-of-shape, the severity of HIIT would discourage new members so much that they probably wouldn't renew their membership.

As an active person and a hard training fighter, wouldn't you rather spend your time on an activity that trims your gut fast and helps your martial arts? So would we. The beauty of HIIT is that it improves your cardio fitness, increases your speed, sharpens your techniques, and trims off that excess baggage in — 15 minutes! If this was an infomercial we would claim three minutes, but it's really 15, and you must admit that is much better then pedaling for 60.

Low intensity training, such as pedaling those nonmoving bicycles, gets its fuel mostly from fat, though the total calories burned are relatively low. HIIT training derives its fuel primarily from carbs and to a lesser degree from fat, but due to its high intensity, the total number of calories burned is much higher than when doing low intensity training.

Here is what this means for your love handles. HIIT burns your body fat up to

50 percent more efficiently than jogging around potholes or pedaling to nowhere. Wait! There is more good news. When you collapse against the wall after your HIIT workout, your body keeps burning calories at an accelerated rate. It's true: Your body keeps burning fat even after you have stopped the exercise. How cool is that?

The only negative is that people who love to spend 60 minutes a workout pedaling lazily to Nowhereville won't like the effort required of HIIT. Yes, it's hard. You sweat and you huff and puff, but you do it for a max of only 15 minutes, and in a month you are leaner, more aerobically fit and your fighting techniques are a little sharper.

Although HIIT can be used in a variety of physical activities, we only discuss shadowsparring, bag work and jogging here. Once you understand the concept using one or all of these three training methods, you can easily apply HIIT to other activities, such as rep practice, kata, sparring, and jumping rope. (It doesn't work with knitting unless you can knit really, really fast.)

How to Start

Understand that this is a tough workout and shouldn't be attempted if you are out of shape, overweight, suffer from orthopedic problems, cardiovascular disease, or haven't exercised for a long time. We strongly advise that you don't do it at all until you have been training for a year and even then you should first get an okay from your doctor.

Start with four minutes Start your first workout with the idea of doing only four minutes of HIIT. That might not seem like much, but if you aren't in the best shape aerobically, you will be calling us nasty names at about minute three. On the other hand, if you are already in good shape aerobically (surprisingly, some overweight people possess good cardiovascular systems) and on the fourth minute feel you can keep going, shoot for five or six minutes. Now, don't kill yourself out of some sense of machismo. If you are hurting at four or five minutes, stop. The idea is to build systematically and sensibly.

To progress If you start your four-minute HIIT on Monday, do it again on Wednesday for four minutes, but on Friday, increase your time to five minutes. In other words, every third session increase your time by one minute, though there are exceptions we talk about in a moment. By the time you reach 15 minutes, several weeks later, it's time to go happily shopping for a new wardrobe.

Shadowsparring

The minimum equipment needed for shadowsparring is a clock with a second hand sweep or a watch with a timer set to beep at 30 second intervals, a water jug and a whole lot of discipline to keep going when you think you might power vomit. Okay, it's not that bad, but almost. Begin by warming up as you usually do before training, doing at least five to 10 minutes of moderate exercise to gradually increase your heartbeat and loosen your joints. HIIT requires a strenuous output, which means injuries are likely when the warm-up is poor, or worse, nonexistent.

Begin shadowsparring at medium speed and continue for 30 seconds. Then for the next 30 seconds, explode as fast and hard as you can as if fighting for your life. Return to medium speed for the next 30-second block, and then explode all-out for another 30. Here is how it looks for four minutes.

- 30 seconds medium speed

- 30 seconds all-out

- 30 seconds medium speed

- 30 seconds all-out

- 30 seconds medium speed

- 30 seconds all-out

- 30 seconds medium speed

- 30 seconds all-out

If your fitness level is average-good and you honestly went all-out every other 30-second block, four minutes is probably enough.

If this is too hard You should be sucking for oxygen after your four-minute session, but if you are absolutely hurting and feel like you are going to blow a heart valve across the room, you need to back off a little and build up to four minutes. Here is an easy way to do that.

The next time you do a HIIT workout, perform the first 30-second, all-out session as hard as you can, but then back off a little on the next three all-out 30-second blasts. Here is how it looks:

• Begin with 30 seconds at medium speed and then do 30 seconds all-out.

• Then do the next 30 seconds at medium speed but do your next all-out 30-second block at 80 or 90 percent. Technically that isn't all-out but let's call it that for now.

• Finish the four-minute session going only 80 to 90 percent in the remaining all-out phases.

• In your next workout, do your first and second all-out 30-second bursts at 100 percent, with your remaining two all-out bursts at 80 to 90 percent.

• On your third workout, which is still only four minutes, add a third 100 percent all-out phase.

• On your fourth workout, go at 100 percent on all four all-out sessions.

• Assess yourself on your fifth workout to see if you are ready to add a minute.

• If not, do another four-minute session of 30-second medium phases

and 30-second all-out phases at 100 percent.

• If on the sixth workout (or the seventh or eighth if you aren't ready) add a minute, to increase your session to five minutes, doing each all-out phase at 100 percent. You are now in condition and in the groove to add one minute every third workout.

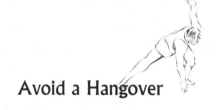

Avoid a Hangover

It's beneficial to stretch after a shadowsparring session. Since your muscles have been contracting incredibly hard and fast, stretching is an important tool to prevent "muscle hangover," a term that refers to that sore and stiff feeling you get in your muscles a day or two after a particularly vigorous training session. Spending five to 10 minutes stretching your arms, shoulders, back and legs not only helps to maintain your flexibility or even progress a little, it also helps eliminate accumulated toxins (from lactic acid). Think of stretching as wringing water from a sponge.

Be careful Since there is no such thing as a Joints-R Us store where you can get replacements, avoid snapping your knees and elbows as you punch and kick in your all-out phase. Some people can snap away for years without a problem, while others begin suffering after just a short while, sometimes to the extent that they are forced to quit training. Unless you absolutely know that your joints are invulnerable and will be so for the rest of your life, always stop your blows two inches short of full extension.

HIIT on the Heavy Bag

HIIT works great when pounding the heavy bag, but be careful. It's important that you monitor your heart rate since working on the big bag can accelerate your pulse into the red zone in a quick hurry. If you find at the start of the third minute of 30 seconds medium and 30 seconds all-out that your heart is threatening to slam its way out of your chest (think of those old Bugs Bunny cartoons when Bugs would see a hot girl bunny and his little red heart would throb out of its furry chest), you might need to remain with four-minute sessions for a few extra workouts. If you feel a need to spend two weeks at each time increment rather than progressing a minute every third workout, so be it. The idea with HIIT is to get lean and healthy, not lean while lying in a coffin. Train smart and in time you will be in peak physical condition.

Be careful Again, you can't go to a Joints R Us store to replace your wrist, elbows, shoulder and knees, so take care to avoid missing the bag with your punches and kicks, especially if your bag swings wildly when struck. You are especially prone to do this near the end of your workout when your techniques are starting to deteriorate. Hyper-extending a knee or elbow ranks near the top of the Things-that-really-hurt list and can take months to heal.

One way to prevent problems is to have a training partner hold the bag so it doesn't swing erratically (he can also encourage you to keep pushing harder when you begin gasping for air). To hold the bag, he should place one arm high and the other arm low and then lean into it to provide optimum control. He needs to be cognizant to keep his arms and body out of your way as you clobber it like a person possessed during the 30-second all-out phases. This is especially important as you become fatigued.

Some people enjoy feeling sore after a good work out. If you are not one of them, do five to 10 minutes of stretching after your session. Pay special attention to stretching your wrists, arms, shoulders, upper and lower back, hips, legs and ankles.

Running

Your primary objective using HIIT is to burn fat at an accelerated rate, while improving your aerobic conditioning for your martial arts training and competing. Know that for some people, the aerobic conditioning gained from running doesn't overlap to sparring, kata or other vigorous martial arts activities. For example, co-author Demeere has used running with great success for years and so have many of his students. On the other hand, it doesn't overlap for Christensen, so he uses shadowsparring and other martial art activities for HIIT. Some of his students say that jogging helps their martial arts, while others say it doesn't. (One of Christensen's early training partners was run over by a car when jogging. After he got out of traction, he joined the group that didn't like it.) If running works for you, great. Just be sure to stretch afterwards since it has a tendency to tighten the leg and back muscles.

For the first 30 seconds simply jog like it's a Sunday afternoon, but then for the next 30 seconds, sprint like you have a pork chop hanging form your back pocket and salivating pit bulls are chasing you. If you haven't sprinted for a while, lower the intensity a little in the all-out phase and follow the progressive system discussed in "Shadowsparring."

A variation   During his competitive years, co-author Demeere ran at a university running track using the same HIIT format just described, though not in 30-second increments. Instead, he sprinted all-out for 300 yards, then walked back to the starting line, and immediately sprinted all-out again. He did this for 10 repetitions. Whether you run on a running track or in a gang infested neighborhood, to use this method you need to establish a starting point and then run all-out for 30 seconds to establish an ending point. Most people find that it helps mentally when they have a set distance to run, especially when fatigue is begging them to cut the HIIT session short.

An option   If you tried HIIT without reading this far, you might be thinking "Yowsa! This is tough!" (snicker, snicker) and if you are in poor condition, you might not have survived to the end of the first four-minute block. If so, refer to the previous segments "Shadowsparring" and "Bag work" to see how to adjust your all-out sessions to progressively build your cardio system, or check out the following methods to help you adapt.

HIIT is a commonly used training device used by track and field competitors who often use a work-to-rest ratio of 1:2, meaning they run all-out for 30 seconds and then run at a moderate pace for two 30-second blocks (one minute). Some use a 1:3 work-to-rest ratio, in that they go all-out for 30 seconds and then run moderately for three, 30-second blocks (90 seconds). Everything we have discussed thus far for shadowsparring, bag work and running has been a 1:1, work-to-rest ratio (30 seconds all-out, 30 seconds moderate).

Let's say you don't feel ready for the 1:1 ratio. Okay, no problem-o. Here is another way for you to get in shape for the 1:1 that usually takes only two or three weeks. Start with a 1:2 work-to-rest ratio for four sets, which means you go all-out for 30 seconds shadowsparring, pounding the bag or running, and then drop to slow to medium speed for 60 seconds. ("Rest" means you go at a moderate pace, not sit in the shade and sip lemonade.) It looks like this for the four sets:

One set of 1:2
One set of 1:2
One set of 1:2
One set of 1:2

Do four sets of the 1:2 ratio for two weeks, and then on the first workout of the third week, replace one 1:2 phase in the middle of your session with a 1:1 phase, 30 seconds all-out followed by 30 seconds at medium speed, like this:

One set of 1:2
One set of 1:2
One set of 1:1
One set of 1:2

Follow this routine for three or four sessions, and then add another 1:1 set:

One set of 1:2
One set of 1:1
One set of 1:1
One set of 1:2

Do that routine for three or four sessions and then add one more 1:1:

One set of 1:2
One set of 1:1
One set of 1:1
One set of 1:1

Do that routine for three or four sessions and then add one more 1:1:

One set of 1:1
One set of 1:1
One set of 1:1
One set of 1:1

Congratulations! You are now doing four sets of 1:1. Do two workout sessions at that pace and then add another minute of 1:1, to increase to five minutes. Keep adding a minute every third workout until you reach 15.

While the 1:2 and 1:3 formulas are an effective way to work toward your ultimate goal of 1:1, you can also use them on those days you want to do HIIT, but for whatever reason your energy is below par. Rather than skip a HIIT workout, do a session of 1:2 or even 1:3. Now don't get lazy and do this all the time, but just on those days when you are dragging but still want to train. If you are like us, you might find that once you are into doing 1:2 or 1:3 that you have more energy than you thought, so you jump to the 1:1 ratio.

It's recommended that you do HIIT training for about eight weeks, three times a week. Longer, say, 12 weeks, and you risk overtraining. When you complete the eighth week, take a couple of weeks off from HIIT and then start again if you choose. You might not be able to start again at 15 minutes and that is okay. You can start at eight or 10 minutes, or you might want to start over at four minutes and progress a minute a week until you again reach 15. In fact, starting at four minutes is recommend by many trainers. We suggest you go by how you feel.

Cardio Split

For years it's been touted that the best and fastest ways to trim the ol' tum-tum is to train aerobically, to get your heart rate up and your lungs puffing. While this is still true, there are recent discoveries that make the effort more convenient, easier and effective.

In the old days, it was believed that you had to go nonstop when training aerobically. Experts said that when you got off the treadmill to take a phone call you would lose all the aerobic training benefit of the exercise. Or, when you had to wait for a traffic light when jogging, you had to run in place so as not to lose your accelerated heart rate.

That is old information; here is what we know now.

Studies show that the more prolonged the aerobic activity the greater the chance you have of mobilizing amino acids and burning muscle. However, people who split their aerobic activity — say half in the morning and half in the evening — burn more fat than people who do it all at once. Remember, cardio workouts speed up your metabolism so that you keep burning fat for a short while after you finish. This means that when you do two cardio sessions, or even three in a day, you burn more calories and fat than in one big aerobic session.

With this in mind, let's look at several ways to spread your aerobics over your day. Find one that fits your life or create one of your own using one of these formats.

Two Sessions for 30 Minutes

Leap out of bed and into your training pants. Shake out the cobwebs with a good five- to 10-minute warm-up, and then shadowspar that sleepy looking person in your bedroom mirror. Duck, bob, weave, punch and kick at a medium pace for 15 minutes. Hit the shower and enjoy the energy shot you just gave yourself. Tonight, do your kata repeatedly for 15 minutes with only 20-second pauses between sets. Both sessions add up to 30 minutes of good cardio for the day.

Two Sessions for 40 Minutes

In the morning, do 20 minutes of leg work: kick the bag, burn reps in the air and practice explosive foot work. Go hard and get your pulse rate up. That evening, do 20 minutes of arm work: punches on the heavy bag and fast reps in the air. Both sessions add up to 40 minutes for the day, and you are looking leaner already.

Three Sessions for 40 Minutes

Park 10 minutes away from work or school and walk as fast as you can (without looking stupid) to your destination, and in the afternoon walk back to your car as fast as you can. That is two sessions and 20 minutes of light aerobics and you even worked your legs a little. That night in class, do your regular workout with the other students, and then hit the heavy bag for 20 minutes after class, for a grand total of 40 minutes of cardio for the day.

Three Sessions for 50 Minutes

At noon, do a fast 20-minute walk, 10 minutes out and 10 minutes back. Before class starts tonight, practice getting up from the floor with speed and finesse for 10 minutes. Lie down on your back and imagine an assailant moving in on you. Get up as fast and as strategically as you can, then plop right down again, this time on your stomach.

Again get up as quickly and strategically as possible. So far you have completed 30 minutes. After class, ask one of the other students to spar, telling him you want to go nonstop at medium speed for 20 minutes. At day's end, you have done 50 minutes of fat-burning aerobics.

Three Sessions for 60 Minutes

Whether you drive or take a bus to work or school, figure out an arrangement where you park your car or get off the bus far enough away that you have to walk 15 minutes to your destination. Now, don't stroll and casually kick stones, but walk fast, as if you just stole something and want to get away quickly without drawing attention by running. On the way back to your car or bus stop in the afternoon, again pour on the speed. That gives you 30 minutes of easy calorie burning aerobics out of the way, and because you walked instead of ran, you saved a little wear and tear on your joints. When you get home, put on your brightly colored spandex running shorts and do 30 minutes of roadwork. That gives you a total of 60 minutes of cardio work for the day, and you can go to bed tonight knowing that you are one fat-burning machine.

Hard Workouts, Easy Workouts

One method to avoid overtraining when splitting your aerobic workouts is to cycle tough sessions with easier ones. If you are a night person, go light in the morning and harder in the evening, or just the opposite if you are an early riser. If you train at mid-day, alter your workouts by training hard one day and then easy the next time. Altering the intensity of your training prevents injuries, burns fat, and gets you in shape fast without the risk of overtraining. Train smart and you will be able to increase the overall intensity of both the light and heavy days in about two weeks.

Dangers of Aerobic Kickboxing

Be careful when participating in aerobic kickboxing. For most people, it improves coordination, strength and cardiovascular health, as it burns 500 to 800 calories an hour, compared to 300 to 400 for a standard aerobics session. But there are hidden dangers since the classes tend to be intense, competitive and designed for people already in excellent condition.

The American Council on Exercise (ACE), a nonprofit organization based in San Diego, issued some advice for prospective aerobic kick boxers. They reported that even basic kickboxing classes require above-average endurance, flexibility and strength. Here are the most common mistakes made by beginners, according to ACE:

• Overextending kicks

• Kicking higher than flexibility allows

• Locking joints when throwing punches or kicking

• Exercising beyond fatigue

• Competing with others

• Wearing weights or holding dumb-bells when throwing punches

• Poor class supervision

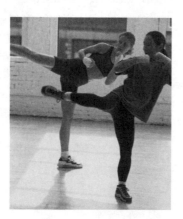

How to Use Fat as Energy in Your Training

If you can grab a handful of your gut and make it jiggle, you need to face the fact that what is jiggling is mostly fat. As we have discussed in earlier chapters, fat contains thousands of calories, so to consider your belly in a positive light, think of it as a large fuel tank hanging around your waist. Thinking even more positively, wouldn't it be great to use that fuel to trim that gut and maybe even get a six-pack of showy ab muscles? It's possible, and here is one way to do it.

Work out Before Breakfast

Tomorrow, get up a little earlier than usual and start your day with a light martial arts workout. Since you haven't eaten carbohydrates for several hours, your body has to get energy from another source: your fat, but only if you train aerobically, which means at moderate to low intensity. Begin with a light warm-up and then go through your forms a few times. Don't go fast or hard, but focus on fluid motions and good form. If your style doesn't have forms or you prefer to shadowspar, great. Just proceed lightly. Want to practice individual techniques, punches and kicks? Go ahead, but do so lightly. Whatever you choose to do, enjoy the nice, easy, flowing movements as you work up a good sweat. When finished, cool off with some light stretches, shower and eat a healthy breakfast. Time: 20 to 30 minutes

If you choose to go hard before breakfast, such as incorporating HIIT, you might find as others have that you are deeply fatigued for the rest of the day. There is no need for that. We suggest that you take it easy, though you should be breathing hard, and enjoy your workout as you burn fat calories. Afterwards, you feel awake and energized for the rest of your day.

For People Severely Overweight

So far we have discussed how to use the martial arts to trim your abdomen, but let's examine briefly how people should train if they are carrying an excessive amount of extra weight. Men carrying over 25 percent body fat and women carrying over 30 percent are considered obese. Know that carrying extra pounds increases the risk of disease and health problems, in particular, problems related to the cardiovascular system (for every pound of fat your body has to supply an extra 200 miles of blood capillaries) and the heart and lungs, which are taxed hard during martial arts training.

Obese people also experience greater stress on their bones and joints. The extra poundage is already forcing them to work hard, so when martial arts training is added to the mix, they become vulnerable to injury. High impact training, such as jumping, board break, hitting the heavy bag, running, and taking hard falls, should be avoided. When a person of average weight runs a few steps, the impact on his ankles is several times his bodyweight, but when an obese person runs or does jump kicks, he overloads his bones and joints to such an extreme that he risks bone breakage and muscle and tendon damage.

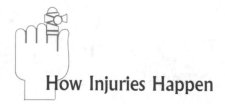

How Injuries Happen

Co-author Demeere knows of a karate school where the teacher routinely made his students team up and take turns piggybacking each other. He made them run about the room, squat and jump, all while carrying the extra weight. By the way, this is an ancient training method that is extremely taxing on the body and potentially injurious. This teacher made children and teenagers do it too, people whose bodies are still developing and vulnerable for injury.

One 17-year-old girl, a regional forms champion, paid the price for her teacher's ignorance when she ripped both knees after being made to run with another student on her back. She subsequently had extensive surgery, but will never be able to train in karate again. This was a healthy girl with previous training and of normal bodyweight. Had she been obese, her injuries might have been even worse.

How to Start Training if You Are Obese

Talk to your doctor first. If he says you can do it, great, but start out slowly, concentrating on the basic kicks, punches and throws. Do kata, as these help you build up your endurance, but don't assume low stances at first. Sinking low places undo pressure on joints and bones in general. Use forms practice to help you get into shape and progressively deepen your stances as you lose weight.

Avoid sparring your first three months of training (we assume here that you train over an hour at least twice a week). During the early months, your body works hard to adapt to the new activity: Your muscles and tendons grow stronger, your bones produce more calcium to grow denser, your endurance increases, and many other good things happen as long as you progress slowly. After three months, you should be reasonably ready for easy sparring. Contact should be light, just taps or touches, and your speed slow to medium. After another two months (it's five months now since you began training), you can step up to a faster pace but the contact should stay light. After more than six months of training and conditioning, begin to slowly increase the contact and let the fun begin.

Our approach is a conservative one because it's so easy to get carried away when sparring. In one exchange you get tapped a little harder than what you agreed to, so you hit back equally hard.

Keep this up and it's likely to cause injury since your body isn't ready for such intensity. There is also a greater risk of taking a bad fall and injuring yourself. While overexertion and falling is all part of the game, your immediate and primary goal is to build a strong, lean and healthy body while having fun and learning something. There is plenty of time for hard play later. Don't risk everything in the early stages of your training.

Choose the Right Teacher

There is a significant social consequence to being obese. Others often stare, make derogatory remarks and go out of their way to make the obese person feel embarrassed or ashamed. This can be especially hard on young children and can impact them for the rest of their lives. Martial arts training, when done systematically, sensibly and in conjunction with a proper eating plan, is an excellent way to overcome obesity (we think it's the best way).

Martial arts is more than just learning how to punch and kick. All good teachers instill basic values in their students: respect for themselves and others, courtesy, etiquette, and a desire to help people. A good teacher doesn't allow obese students to be insulted or emotionally hurt in their classes. He creates a positive environment that encourages everyone to strive to be the best he can be, and he sets a tone that makes everyone eager to put on their uniform and travel the path toward a healthier, leaner, stronger and better human being.

Develop powerful abs with crunches and kicks

Say you have followed one or more of the fat reduction plans discussed in this book and now your abs are starting to peek through. Well, peek is all they are going to do if you haven't done ab exercises in conjunction with the fat trimming. Even if you don't care about a visible six-pack, you still need to do the exercises because powerful abs are a must for powerful punches, kicks and grappling.

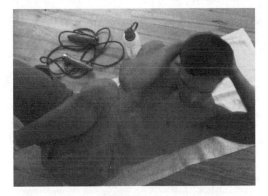

There are many effective ab exercises (and not just a few potentially harmful ones) that can be found in books and magazines. The ones discussed here are particularly beneficial for the specific needs of martial artists.

Tips to Optimize Your Ab Exercises

Here are some general tips that make each rep as productive as possible:

- Pull in your stomach on each rep as if you were trying to touch your bellybutton to your spine. Too many martial artists push theirs out when doing crunches, which over time can result in a protruding gut even when it's strong and lean.

- Maintain good back support throughout the exercise. Don't engage in exercises that put undue pressure on your spine, especially if you already have back problems.

- Don't hold your breath. Breathe out as you contract your abs to make it easier to pull in your abdominal muscles and increase the intensity of the rep.

- Don't exercise your abs on a hard surface. The discomfort can be distracting and you want your mind to focus on your abs.

- Use good technique. Just as good form is important when executing a martial arts move, it's also important when exercising. It's of little value to your ab muscles when you swing your legs or upper-body to finish those last few difficult reps. It's potentially dangerous whenever you contort yourself forcefully. Lower the number of reps until you can do more with good form.

- The function of your primary abdominal muscles is to bring your upper body and pelvis together. In other words, they help you to curl into a ball. If an exercise doesn't allow you to bring your lower and upper halves together, you are probably using your legs to raise your trunk

- Stretch your abs after exercising to reduce soreness and help keep a strong yet flexible midsection.

- If any ab exercise in your class hurts your back, discuss it with your instructor and ask if you can do a different one in its place. You will thank us for this tip when you get older.

Here are some highly effective ab exercises that strengthen the abdominal region in record time.

Swiss Ball Crunch

A Swiss ball is a big, durable and versatile piece of equipment that, depending on size and material, can generally be bought for under $40. There are two major advantages to using a ball: It conforms to the shape of your back to provide excellent support and, since it's an unstable platform, your abs have to work extra hard to maintain your balance while exercising. This makes for a challenging and safe workout.

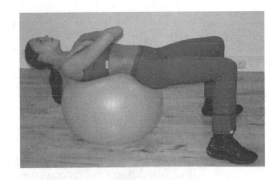

Lie on the ball so your lower and middle back are supported and your upperbody is angled slightly above horizontal. Plant your feet firmly on the floor and keep your knees bent. Cross your arms over your chest with your elbows held tightly against your body.

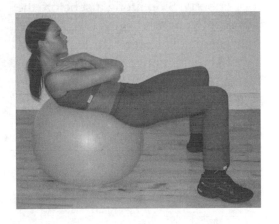

Slowly curl your upper body by lifting your shoulders and upper back toward your lower body while exhaling and pulling in your gut. Return to the starting position and do another rep.

Do 3 sets, 15 reps

To increase the difficulty, push with your feet and "walk" backwards until the ball is centered under your lower spine. This stretches your abs as you lower your upper body to the starting position. With the added range of motion your abs are forced to work harder.

Swiss Ball Reverse Crunch

Lie down and center your back on the ball. Grab hold of a doorpost, kitchen table or have a partner hold your arms as you perform the exercise.

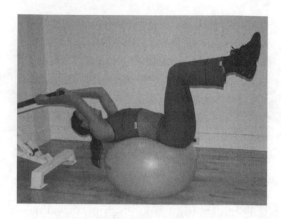

Keep your legs together and raise them slowly, using your hip muscles. Don't cheat and use momentum by swinging them up. (Yes, we know it's harder and it hurts your ab muscles when you do it correctly.) Continue to lift your legs slowly until your knees are over your upper body. Stop lifting just before the tension in your abs begins to lessen and immediately lower your legs slowly. Make your abs work continuously throughout the set and don't give them a rest break between the reps.

Do 3 sets, 15 reps

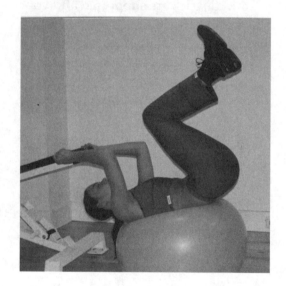

Reverse Trunk Twist

Reverse trunk twists on the ball are hard, but produce amazing results. If your abs are out of shape, start out on the floor and in a couple of weeks you should be ready for the ball. (Avoid these entirely if you have lower back problems.) For now, do them on the floor.

Lie on your back with your body straight and your arms spread to the side, though you might want to hold onto something as you did in the Swiss ball reverse crunch. Raise your straightened legs until they are pointing straight up— consider this the starting position—then lower them slowly to your left side.

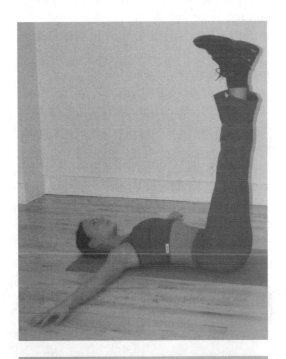

Keep your knees locked and your legs together throughout this movement. Don't raise your opposite shoulder when your feet touch the floor and don't stop to rest (cursing and groaning is okay). Raise your legs slowly back to the starting position and then lower them slowly to the right side. Never, at any stage in the exercise, swing or suddenly drop your legs. Doing so is potentially injurious to your back.

Do 2 sets, 10 reps

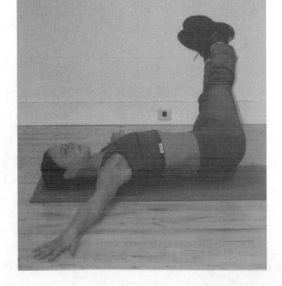

Slow Motion Shadowboxing Using Only Kicks

Since the abs are so instrumental in delivering explosive, pile driving leg attacks, you can use your kicks to develop your midsection.

First do a warm-up and some light stretching. Once you are ready, begin shadowsparring with only your legs, but go s-l-o-w-l-y. Flow from one kick to another without relying on momentum, using every kick you know or just four or five of your favorites. You want your muscles to work hard in every phase of each painfully slow kick — the chamber, the launch, the retraction, and the return to the floor. If you normally target your opponent's legs, strive to kick as high as your flexibility allows in this exercise to force your abs, front and sides, to work overtime. This strengthens the specific ab muscles needed for awesome kicking power.

Do 3 rounds, 5 minutes each

Machine Gun Kicks

As the name suggests, this exercise involves rapid fire kicking done against a heavy bag. We suggest you do them with a partner so you can take turns catching your breath while the other fires his salvo at the bag. First, do a good warm-up and stretch to avoid injuries. To focus on your ab and oblique muscles, use only the sidekick, roundhouse and spinning kicks. Let's begin with 10 left leg roundhouse kicks and then 10 with your right leg.

Concentrate on exploding with each kick, driving from your hips rather than just snapping from your knees. Don't wait until the last three reps to go hard, but go all-out from your first rep to your last. The operative word is explode. As you retract your leg after each kick, snap your foot back to your starting position, but rather than set it down gently, bounce it off the floor and right back into another kick. Think of your foot as a rubber ball: The harder you throw it down, the harder it bounces back up. Too many fighters use the bounce to do all the work rather than lifting the kick with their hips. The bounce gives you speed while incorporating the hips gives you power as you try to kick through the bag. Remember, go hard from the very beginning so that the first whack! is as loud as the last.

Rear leg roundhouse: 2 set, 10 reps

Sidekick: 2 sets, 10 reps

Any spinning kick: 2 sets, 10 reps

When these become easy for you, increase your reps to 15 or 20 and your sets to three or four. You can change kicks, too. For example, try your roundhouses with your lead leg, your sidekicks with your rear leg and any other spinning kicks you like. Just limit your kicks to these particular ones since they involve your ab muscles more than, say, scoop kicks or stomps. Consider incorporating machine gun kicking into the HIIT workout discussed earlier to develop killer abs, killer kicks and killer lungs.

Fast Facts

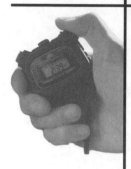

- It's one thing to reduce your weight to fit into a pair of slacks, but it's a whole other arena when you do it to go up against fighters trying their hardest to kick and punch you in the face.

- If you have to consistently train hard and diet hard to stay in a given division, it might be time to move up to the next one.

- Too many fighters underestimate the time they need to trim off the pounds.

- If you plan your training cycle well and follow it, you will always be in good shape, within a pound or two of your weight class.

- It's recommended that a competitive fighter have less than 15 percent body fat.

- If you are naturally lean with minimal fat, it's going to be hard for you to lose weight without losing precious muscle.

- Dropping 300 calories a day is so insignificant that you won't feel a thing and, more importantly, it won't interfere with your health, energy to train or your metabolism.

- If you have to train at a great intensity and restrict your calories up to the day of the competition, you have probably reached a stage where you should move up to a higher weight division.

- Zigzagging is an excellent way to add quality muscle that ultimately helps your fighting. Fat weight won't help at all.

- If you get anxious and gain too quickly, you get unwanted fat. If you lose too quickly, you lose valuable muscle.

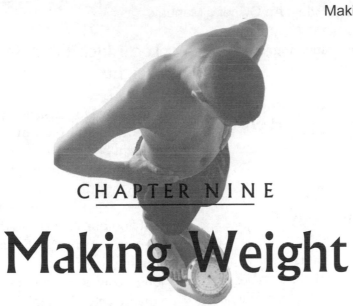

CHAPTER NINE

Making Weight

Making weight for competition is a piece of cake (pun intended) or a nightmare depending on in which weight division you want to fight, your current weight and the time you have to achieve the desired weight. Your current weight and the date of the competition are a given but at what weight you enter should be a matter of careful consideration.

Diet Down the Right Way

Too often, fighters diet to such an extreme that they end up as mere ghosts of themselves on competition day. The fast weight loss, drastic calorie reduction and overtraining leaves them drained and so listless that they have to dig deeply into their reserves to find whatever is left to bring to the fight. It's one thing to reduce your weight to fit

into a pair of slacks, but it's a whole other arena when you do it to go up against fighters trying their hardest to kick and punch you in the face. Clearly, it's in the best interest of your facial features to do it right.

Many times a fighter, amateur or professional, wants to remain in his weight category though his body type dictates he should move up. Such a fighter would do well to think about his health rather than a contractual obligation, a desire to defend a title, or concern about facing a particular fighter in the next higher weight division. While these reasons are all valid in the fight game, they nonetheless lead to potential health concerns. Dieting below one's optimal fight weight exhausts the body's reserves, depletes essential vitamins and minerals and, when done repeatedly for several years, exposes the fighter to increased risk of various injuries. Weakened bones, for example, aren't something you want in the fighting arts

How can you decide which weight division is right for you? Here are some considerations.

What is Your Body Type?

As discussed in Chapter 2, "Somotypes," certain body types are more prone to store fat than others. For them, dieting is relatively easy because they have more to lose. However, if you are naturally lean with minimal fat, it's going to be hard for you to lose weight without losing precious muscle. Revisit "Somotypes" so you know in which category you fit.

Critique Your Diet

If you have been overindulging or eating poorly for several months or years, it's likely you are packing around lots of body fat, even if you are naturally inclined to be lean. Eat poorly long enough and those dreaded love handles encircle your waist like a not-so-loving boa constrictor. Now, if you have been training hard and eating healthily, but you have acquired some minor love handles over the last two or three years, though you have gained only a pound or two, that just might be your natural state. Can you change it? Yes. Is it hard to maintain that change? Yes. Read on.

Too Much Effort to Make Weight

If you have to consistently train hard and diet hard to stay in a given division, it might be time to move up to the next one. In Chapter 10, we discuss how to cycle your training prior to competition. One aspect of cycling your workouts is that you burn fewer calories as you near the tournament day; though you are training hard, you aren't training as long. Now, if during this phase you find you are actually gaining weight, though you are eating healthily and controlling your calorie intake, your body might be sending you a message that it feels best and functions best a little heavier. In other words, if you have to train at a great intensity and restrict your calories up to the day of the competition, you have probably reached a stage where you should move up to a higher division.

Do You Gravitate Toward One Weight?

While there is some discussion as to the scientific basis of this concept, it appears that fighters tend to gravitate towards a certain ideal weight, meaning they know they compete at their best when they have a specific ratio of muscle and body fat. Empirical evidence suggests that while the ratio stays the same, the body weight rarely does.

Co-author Demeere began competing at 183 pounds, a comfortable weight where his perfect ratio of muscle to fat supplied him with lots of endurance and power. Over the next five years he trained with weights, increasing his muscle mass to 192 pounds, still with the same ratio of fat to muscle. He felt comfortable with the increased weight and when he moved up to the next weight division, he happily found he had tremendous strength, explosiveness and endurance to meet the heavier competitors.

Know what weight works best for you and be prepared to go higher if doing so is a natural evolution.

A Diet and Training Plan That Works for You

Finding which weight division is best for you is the easy part. The hard part begins as you work to ensure that you make the weight with energy and motivation to fight once you get there. It's especially hard if you have allowed your weight to increase because of poor training habits or lax eating. Solution: Don't do that to yourself. Whether you want to gain weight or lose, you need to find a diet and training schedule that works for you using any one of the many approaches presented in this book.

Start Early to Make Weight

Too many fighters underestimate the time they need to trim off the pounds. They believe that all they have to do is increase their training sessions some and the flab melts away. Unfortunately, they discover too late that while that is a good start, it's really not that simple. It's not complicated, but it's a tad more involved than just increasing training. The best insurance against still being overweight on tournament day is to start out early. Now, if you approach the task too conservatively, you come in too heavy, and if you hit it too aggressively, you risk being exhausted and over trained. What is needed, therefore, is a plan somewhere in the middle. Here are two that work great:

Lose one pound a week   Say a tournament is 10 weeks off and you are 10 pounds heavier than what your weight class allows. While you could use the plan in Chapter 10 to lose 10 pounds in 21 days, the good news is that there is no need to put yourself through that tough regimen during a time when you should be focusing on polishing your tournament techniques. A much easier way, one that is virtually effortless, is to calculate a weight loss formula that trims one pound per week. This might seem too conservative, but you have 10 weeks to accomplish it, so why kill yourself? Remember, whenever you strive to lose more than one pound a week you also risk losing some of your hard-earned muscle.

Dropping a pound of fat per week means you need to cut and burn 3,500 calories every seven days. Here are a few pointers to help you along the way in calculating the right formula for you:

- You need to have a clear idea of what your body needs during the 10-week period. Calculate the right ratio of carbs, protein and fat for you (refer to Chapter 3) and how many calories you need each day if you were to maintain your current weight. Be especially cognizant of getting enough protein to help minimize muscle mass loss, which occurs even with conservative weight reduction plans such as this one. Don't get lazy and attempt to guesstimate your calories and percentages because you might discover during your, say, sixth week that you overate a few hundred calories each day. Do it right. Preparation is half the battle

- Look for easy-to-cut calories. Do we really need to say that you have no business eating junk food and candy? Good. If you normally eat a lot of it, just cutting them out of your diet will eliminate thousands of calories a week. But if you just have to have a little junk so you won't go stark raving mad, choose one or two (not three) items to have on your Dirt Day.

- Watch for hidden calories. Use calorie-free sweetener in your coffee instead of the real stuff. Eliminate butter on your bread. Gravy is evil and so is sour cream. These calorie monsters are used to enhance the taste of your food, but they have to go. Hey, stop sobbing and stay disciplined for the 10 weeks you need to prepare yourself for competition. Once you bring back the gold, then you can take your tastebuds out on the town.

- If you use a training cycle (Chapter 10) to prepare for your competition, your increased training and conservative calorie reduction will melt away unwanted pounds. Since you have to prepare for the competition anyway, use the training cycle approach to do it systematically and come out at the end 10 pounds lighter and ready to fight.

- Increase your calorie-burning aerobic and anaerobic work: sparring, all-out drills, bag work, non-stop kata and so on. These are good preparation for your competition, anyway, so add a little more, cut out some unnecessary calories and be a lean, mean, 10-pounds lighter fighting machine on the day of the tournament.

Stay in shape so you don't have to lose
Arguably the best approach is to ensure that you don't need to lose weight, or at least not much. If you plan your training cycle well and follow it, you will always be in good shape, within a pound or two of your weight class. This makes life so much easier and allows you to focus on your fighting techniques and strategy, as opposed to being distracted by having to trim off some extra jiggly stuff. This takes

discipline and planning, but you can do it.

Determine your ideal weight: Begin by measuring your body fat percentage. It's recommended that a competitive fighter have less than 15 percent. Now, some fighters feel comfortable carrying more, but they should know it's useless weight that slows and inhibits their mobility, and decreases their overall effectiveness. "Sure, I got a belly, but I'm really fast," some argue. Great, but how much faster would they be without the tummy to lug around? Extra weight is something you want your opponent to have, not you.

Seven percent body fat is as low as you should go. Lower, and you risk serious health problems. Yes, competitive bodybuilders often drop to three or four percent, but they remain there for only a few days, sometimes only the day of the contest. Carrying 15 percent is comfortable and easy to maintain.

Determine a buffer zone: Figure out how much buffer zone you want on either side of your ideal weight. For example, if your ideal weight is 150 pounds, your buffer zone should be no more than five pounds divided evenly. This means you can go up to 152.5 pounds or down to 147.5 pounds. The trick, meaning the real effort, is to stay within those those boundaries for the entire competitive season. To do so, carefully monitor your weight by checking the scales at least once a week. If the needle indicates you are nearing the upper or lower edge of your buffer zone, take immediate steps to increase your training and count calories to get back on course, a relatively easy task since you need to adjust only a pound or two. Never allow yourself to go beyond your zone. Once the competitive phase is over, you can rest, recuperate and allow your buffer zone to expand a little more. But be careful. We are talking 10 pounds at the most, five pounds on either side of your ideal weight. Should you make it 20 pounds, you are in for a lot of extra effort next season to get back into your weight division.

The Zigzag Diet

Lets look at another conservative eating plan used by fighters, one that is easy to follow, relatively nonrestrictive and fits nicely into your lifestyle. You can use it to maintain your weight, drop a couple of pounds should your weight be nudging too close to the upper edge of your buffer zone, or to gain quality muscle should you want to move into the next division or the top edge of your current one.

When you zigzag your calorie intake, you systematically and conservatively change the number of calories you consume to "confuse" your metabolism into not overreacting. Whenever you diet too fast and too extreme (as in a crash diet), your body reacts by slowing your metabolism: conserving calories, sodium, holding water, and more. With this diet, however, just as your metabolism determines that you have changed what you usually feed it and starts to adapt to the new calorie intake, you switch back to eating your normal amount. Zigzagging works whether you are trying to lose or gain weight.

It's rather like the fighting concept called broken rhythm. You throw a backfist and your opponent blocks it. You throw another and he blocks it again. Now he has you figured out, or so he thinks. You fake a third backfist and as he goes for the block, you kick him in the groin. Same thing happens here (except there is no groin kicking). Just as your metabolism begins to adapt because it thinks you are going to feed it, say, less calories, you return to eating your usual amount for two days. Your metabolism relaxes, thinking all is well, and then you again reduce the number for another five days.

When using the zigzag diet to add muscle, you benefit by gaining less fat than with other methods. This is because when zigzagging, you increase your caloric intake for a few days and then drop back to your normal intake for two days. Think of it as taking two steps forward and one step back. Continuing in this fashion for 10 weeks provides you with the necessary calories to gain muscle with the barest minimum of fat.

Your body requires a negative energy balance to lose weight and a positive one to gain muscle. Whichever plan you follow, you must proceed conservatively. If you get anxious and gain too quickly, you get unwanted fat. If you lose too quickly, you lose valuable muscle. The cornerstone of the zigzag diet is the sensible way in which it helps you stay within your weight division, or gradually drop to the next lowest or move up to the next highest.

Here is how it works in detail:

To lose weight Say you want to lose weight because you are near the upper edge of your buffer zone:

- First calculate your daily calorie requirements to maintain your present weight using one of the formulas explained in Chapter 3.

- Then for five days eat two calories less per pound of your bodyweight. For example, if you weigh 150 pounds, cut 300 calories each day. You can easily do this by eliminating butter on your bread, eating one or two fewer cookies and replacing regular milk with skim.

- For the next two days, eat the number of calories you need to maintain your weight.

- Then go another five days eating 300 calories under your maintenance requirement.

- Zigzag for three weeks and you will be one pound lighter.

Dropping 300 calories a day is so insignificant that you won't feel a thing and, more importantly, it won't interfere with your health, energy to train or your metabolism.

To gain weight You want to move up a weight division because you are close to its boundaries and believe you can easily handle the extra pounds of muscle. Since you have already added some lean mass through weight training and you want to continue pumping the weights, you feel dieting down would be too hard and too debilitating on your energy. In other words, all indications are your body wants to be heavier.

- Add two calories per pound of bodyweight. So, if you weigh 150 pounds, add 300 calories each day for five days. (No, you don't get to do it with cookies. Read "Important tips" below)

- Then for two days eat your normal calorie intake to maintain your weight.

- Continue zigzagging for three weeks and *tuh duh,* you are the proud owner of at least one more pound of muscle.

Important Tips for Losing or Gaining

- The zigzag diet assumes you eat at least five small meals every day.

- Cut or add the 300 calories evenly among your three main meals, 100 calories at each.

- When adding calories to gain weight, make sure they are from protein and complex carbs, never from fat.

- When adding calories to gain weight, increase your resistance work, weight training or dynamic tension (see Chapter 11)

- When you want to lose weight, cut calories from fat, not from protein or carbs.

When you don't reach your goal
Whether striving to gain or lose, you should see results in three weeks, but since the human body sometimes has a mind of its own, you just might not get them. After you finish swearing and sweeping up the lamp you threw against the wall, add another 100 calories if you are trying to gain, or subtract another 100 if you are trying to lose. So if you weigh 150 pounds, follow the same procedure as before but add or subtract 400 calories.

When you don't lose Resist the temptation to just cut calories every day, especially if you aren't losing as quickly as you would like. If you only do the down-zag, that is, if you drop calories every day, your metabolism slows and reacts as it does when you crash diet, though to a lesser degree. It's the up-zag, normal eating, that prevents this from happening. Think of zigzagging as a lie you tell your body. "I'm not really dieting, so there is no need for you to drastically re-set my metabolism."

When you don't gain   Resist the temptation to add the extra calories every day. The down-zag (normal calorie intake) helps you burn off any excess fat you might accumulate during the up-zag (300 or 400 calorie increase). Omit the normal eating days from the plan and you risk gaining weight that is largely fat. Zigzagging allows your body to change its muscle-to-fat-ratio without the side effects of gaining too much fat, as usually happens when you force-feed every day. Remember, this diet is meant to work over the long haul, gradually.

Zigzagging requires that you do a little math, but it's not hard math even for math-challenged guys like us; it's worth the effort to find a pencil and pad. If you use zigzag eating throughout your fighting career, you won't have to go through the painful process of having to make weight up or down, for competition. [27] [28]

Zigzagging to Gain Muscle vs. Other Methods

There is good news, bad news, and good news with zigzagging. The first good news is that you will gain weight with the program. The bad news is that it takes a little longer than other methods, but the second good news is that your weight gains are mostly quality punching and kicking muscle. In contrast, other programs designed to increase your weight more quickly usually accumulate lots of fat with the muscle gain — fat that slows you down and makes you breathe harder. Zigzagging is an excellent way to add quality muscle that ultimately helps your fighting. Fat weight won't help at all.

Last Minute Tricks

Co-author Demeere once attended a world championship competition where an entire fighting team had erred when pre-registering, resulting in every member of the team placed into a division lower than their fighting weight. The organizing committee steadfastly refused to let the team change their entry, which meant that each fighter had to shed at least eight pounds in just a few days. Amazingly, all succeeded in dropping the weight — a result of jogging and working out in plastic training suits and other gimmicks — but it came at a cost, a big one. Drained of power, endurance and energy, every last fighter was soundly defeated in the competition.

Most weigh-in problems aren't as extreme. Usually it's just a matter of dropping a pound or two, and with an improvised training session a fighter can sweat off enough fluids to make weight. However, if the difference is more than two pounds, the task becomes harder, more complicated and usually more debilitating.

One pound of fat equals 3,500 calories, far too many to burn off in just a few hours or even a few days before a competition. Now, you can easily lose a few pounds of fluid weight, but you will experience what the team discovered: You make weight, but you are too drained to lift your arms to fight. Since your body is mostly water, it just makes sense that you can't function without it, let alone fight well in competition.

But can't you just drink some water or a sports drink after the weigh-in to rehydrate? Nope. It takes a while for your body to recover from the dehydration you inflicted, anywhere from one to several days, depending on how much was lost and your constitution. Along with the lost fluids, you lose power and endurance, which also takes a while to get back.

Even more extreme   If training in special suits or taking long saunas to lose precious fluids are not bad enough (in extreme cases, performing intense exercise while super-dehydrated causes death), some competitors take laxatives and diuretics to drop even more pounds. Not only do these cause significant dehydration, they can also cause profound intestinal problems. Also, certain laxatives and diuretics are banned as a doping product. So if you were to use them and win your match but then were to test positive, you lose, maybe more than the match. For the professional fighter, losing this way can mean a lack of income since few sponsors pay for a banned athlete.

One last, nagging thought   Along with your debilitating physical condition from rapid weight loss and the mental stress of worrying about making weight and then trying to compete when you feel like crud, is that little taunting voice in the back of your head going, "I told you so, I told you so. None of this would have happened if you had prepared yourself better and monitored your weight. Neener, neener, neener."

Fast Facts

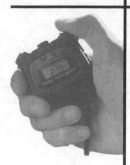

- There can be any number of situations where you need to lose weight quickly, so understanding that reality, we reluctantly decided to add this chapter to show you the safest way we know to drop weight fast.

- While some people have a naturally fast metabolism and lose weight easily, others have to fight for every ounce lost.

- If you normally don't push yourself in your workouts, the sudden increased workload in this program puts you at risk of injury and overtraining. Proceed carefully.

- To lose weight fast, you have to eat more often than the typical three-meals-a-day system. We suggest five or six meals to turn your body into a state-of-the-art, calorie-burning engine.

- After the 10-day training phase, expect your fellow students to be surprised at your improved fitness, the quality of your techniques and your trimmer body.

- If you did an extra 30 minutes of bag work today and then later gave into that piece of candy, you just destroyed the calorie burning benefits of the bag work.

- If you normally do, say, three sets of 20 reps each of basic punches and kicks, increase to six sets of 20 reps. Or, remain at three but double your reps to 40 per set.

- When you do a One-Minute Training sessions two, three, four or more times a day, in conjunction with your calorie cutting and the extra hard training sessions, the mini-workouts help keep your metabolism stoked like a red-hot furnace.

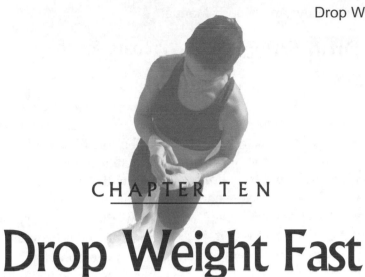

C H A P T E R   T E N

Drop Weight Fast

Your authors believe firmly in making healthy lifestyle changes regarding diet, but neither of us believes in quick-fix solutions. It's a far better plan and far easier to stay in condition year round so that you never have to suffer through a quick and strenuous weight loss program. Nonetheless, there can be any number of situations where you need to lose weight quickly, so understanding that reality, we reluctantly decided to add this chapter to show you the safest way we know to drop weight fast. Understand that it's hard on your body and that you should never do it more than once a year. And it's especially important to get plenty of sleep during these regimens since your body is working so hard for you.

There is no gimmick and there is no magic bullet to quick weight loss (those you find in late-night infomercials and in magazine ads). The reality is it's hard work since you have to cut back on the chow a little and train hard, very hard.

Whether you just want to look good at the beach, look all slim and trim for that special function or make the middleweight division at the big tournament in 10 or 21 days, it can be done — with effort. In the end, when you reach your weight loss goal, you will be slimmer and your martial arts will have improved, too. Life is good. (It would be even better if there were no calories in pizza.)

Warning

It's hard on your body any time you drop weight quickly. Dropping it in a hurry to make weight for competition by increasing your training load and cutting calories carries an even greater risk. With our plan, you drop pounds as healthily as possible, but still you might end up so drained on competition day that a turtle could beat you to the punch. Don't say we didn't warn you. (Refer to Chapter 9 as to the best way to make weight for competition.)

How to Drop 5 Pounds in 10 Days

First the bad news: One pound of fat equals 3,500 calories. That means to dump five pounds, you have to eliminate from your diet and burn up in training a total of 17,500 calories — and do so in 10 days. This takes willpower and sweat, but the good news is that you are going to be one happy camper on that 10th day when it's all over, and the mirror reflects a leaner you.

Warning   If you normally don't push yourself in your workouts, the sudden increased workload in this program puts you at risk of injury and overtraining. If you have a medical condition, a cold, flu or you don't know about your health, we advise you to first see a doctor. This isn't the time to play macho.

Navy SEALS

Should you start whimpering the third day into the program, think about our poor Navy SEALS in a training phase called "Hell Week." It's aptly named because for five and a half days the SEALS train virtually nonstop, though they do manage to slip in four hours of sleep. That is not four hours a night, but four hours spread over the five and a half days. During this hellish week, trainees burn up to 7000 calories per day. Compared to that, our program is a piece of cake, a moist, rich, chocolate cake with a rainbow of sprinkles on top and a scoop of ice cream on the side.

Prepare for It

Those who have problems with this program usually fail because they approach it haphazardly. If you plan on starting this 10-day effort tomorrow, please take the time right now to sit down with a notebook and lay out your schedule for the next week and three days. Write down every workout you plan to do and schedule them into your week so you don't forget and accept other appointments during your training time. Consider your notebook a stone tablet on which you can't scratch out your workouts for a hot date or a movie. Your schedule is permanent; it will happen. Besides writing down your training schedule, also note a general idea of what you will eat for each meal and what time you will go to bed. To reiterate, you must schedule in lots of rest.

If your notebook looks intimidating, keep reminding yourself that this rigid schedule lasts only 10 days. If it helps, each night put an X over the completed day in your calendar. Or, count the days as they do in the army: If you have five to go, don't say, "I have five more days," but say, "I have four days and a wake-up." Yes, you still have to diet and train on that last wake-up day, but calling it that sounds better than saying "five days."

When you finish putting all your notations into your notebook, look at it, grit your teeth, tighten your resolve and prepare to unleash your powerful discipline for the coming 10-day period. (Refer to Chapter 14, "Getting your head on right.")

Eat Frequent Meals

You were given a teaser on this concept in Chapter 1; now let's look at it closer. To lose weight fast, you have to eat more often than the typical three-meals-a-day system. We suggest five or six meals: a small one every three to four hours. This proven principle turns your body into a state-of-the-art, calorie-burning engine, as opposed to the slow calorie-burning engine that gets fueled three times a day. The extra meals significantly increase your metabolism causing you to burn more calories even when resting. Is there a catch? Of course. Your meals need to be smaller than those you eat only three times a day.

Better for overall health   Studies have shown that a common American "gorging" diet, in which a person gets all of his daily calories in three meals a day (or worse: one or two meals a day), may lead to higher levels of LDL, or "bad" cholesterol than when following an eating plan where calories are divided among multiple meals throughout the day.

A study published in the British Medical Journal determined blood concentrations of "bad" and total cholesterol decreased steadily as the number of meals eaten per day increased. Cholesterol levels were much lower in people eating six-or-more meals than in those eating only one or two. This finding has been supported by other studies, as well. When you eat five or six daily meals, your body converts less from the food into fat and

you maintain a constant blood-sugar level, which keeps your energy on a constant level. [29]

In a nutshell, frequent meals provide the following benefits:

- They increase calorie consumption because your body stays busy digesting food.

- Your energy levels stays even throughout the day, meaning you don't get sudden peaks and debilitating valleys.

- You don't suffer from hunger.

- Frequent meals might lower your bad cholesterol.

- Eating frequently gives you pleasure and something to look forward to.

Plan Your Meals

Depending on your job or school schedule, it can be challenging to fit in all the meals during your day. To work around this, you need to be organized by preparing your meals before you go to work, putting them in air-sealed lunchboxes to keep them fresh and knowing exactly what you will eat at each meal. If it's exceptionally awkward for you to eat a small meal, consider concealing a couple of energy bars in your pocket to munch on at mid-morning and mid-afternoon. If your boss or teacher is strict about eating, break little pieces off in your pocket discreetly and nonchalantly pop them in your mouth. Consider this good stealth practice. Consider it — ninja eating.

Cut Calories

This is the rough part because you need to cut at least 500 to 600 calories a day for the next 10 days. An irony here is that if you normally eat a lot of junk food, cutting calories will be a piece of cake (pun intended), since eliminating one milkshake can reduce your calorie intake as much as 1000 calories. It's no more sweets for you and don't even think about soft drinks or alcohol. And high-fat foods? Forget about it - they carry the plague. Kiss these goodies goodbye right now and instantly cut hundreds of calories from your day.

Now, if you already eat a healthy, calorie conscious diet, it's going to be tougher for you to cut an extra 600 than it is for the junk food addict. But hey! You laugh in the face of tough, right? You must find those calories right now and kill them with extreme prejudice. You can do it.

Christensen, for example, is a peanut butter junkie and eats it as if there will soon be a shortage. Though peanut butter is good for you (it contains protein and the good oil), it's calorie dense. So when he needs to drop a couple of pounds, he reduces two of his daily servings by half, so that he still

enjoys his fix, but with 200 fewer calories. This nearly inconsequential sacrifice trims nearly two pounds a month.

Are you eating healthy bread, but three slices of it? Cut back to one, say, half a slice with two of your meals. Do you drink milk to satisfy your thirst? Drink water instead when you are thirsty and enjoy a half glass of milk with two of your five or six meals. Watch out for those sneaky bites when you cook or clean up the table after your family because every little one contains calories.

Students often moan that they can't possibly cut back any further. "Oh yeah," we ask, in an annoyingly smug tone. "Then how did you gain four pounds over the last two months?" Never think that you can't cut back somewhere because every little bite adds up.

Increase Training

The real kicker of this program (yup, another pun) is that you have to turn up the intensity of your training a notch by doing something physical every day. If you normally train two or three times a week, doing something every day might seem daunting, but keep in mind that you only have to do this for 10 days. Rather, nine days and a wake-up.

Before you even consider what you are going to do, know that you are going to do a lot of it. If you normally work out for one hour, tack on another 30 minutes, or 45. Expect to do some huffing and puffing because most of it is going to be aerobic to get those ugly calories burning at an accelerated rate. Here are three methods that we like. If you favor other aerobic martial arts training methods, do those instead.

HIIT   High intensity interval training eats calories like a ravenous teenager. Refer to "HIIT" in Chapter 8 and follow the procedure using whatever training regimen you want: shadowsparring, jogging or bag work. Within a couple of days your fat will scream, "I'm melllltiiiing!"

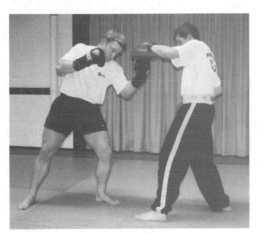

Increase speed and power   Punching and kicking hard and fast burns more calories than punching and kicking at medium speed. This is because it takes additional calories to contract your muscles more forcefully. After a good warm-up, proceed through your normal number of sets and reps, but go all-out on every rep. Make sure they are fast and powerful to maximize calorie consumption. It's safest to go all-out on a heavy bag, partner-held pads or kicking shields. It's more risky when shadowsparring since it's so easy to overextend your joints, thus making a scene when you collapse on the floor and thrash about in pain (though thrashing will burn a few extra calories).

Double your sets and reps   If you normally do, say, three sets of 20 reps each of basic punches and kicks, increase to six sets of 20 reps. Or, remain at three sets but double your reps to 40 per set. If one day you are oozing energy, double your sets and reps.

Here is how the options look:

- Double your sets from 3 to 6 sets x 20 reps

- Do your usual 3 sets, but double your reps from 20 to 40

- Double your sets form 3 to 6 and also your reps from 20 to 40

Improve your endurance and skills   A wonderful benefit to all your efforts is that as you melt fat and lower your body weight, your cardiovascular system improves so you can train even harder and longer. By doing HIIT, extra sets and reps, and hammering out punches and kicks faster and harder than you do normally, your techniques improve from all the extra work. After the 10-day training phase, expect your fellow students to be surprised at your improved fitness, the quality of your techniques and your trimmer body. **Note:** Check the end of this chapter for trouble shooting tips.

How to Drop 10 Pounds in 21 Days

We want to mention again that losing weight fast — and 10 pounds in 21 days is fast — is not the preferred way to drop excess pounds, but if you absolutely must, we want to show you how to do it as safely as possible. Now, if you thought losing five pounds in 10 days was tough, dropping 10 pounds in three weeks — a pound every other day — will really get you moaning. For this, you have to be even stricter with your diet and you must train even longer and harder. Again, we strongly advise you to check with your doctor to ensure you have no hidden problems before beginning the rigors that are to come.

A Warm-up Reminder

We want to underscore this and lecture you like your mother: Learn from our errors and never skip the warm-up. Always begin with jumping jacks, light stretching, and arm and knee rotations. When you finish training, be sure to cool down with more light stretching. We didn't follow this advice in our early days and we paid with serious injuries. Always, always, always do a warm-up. Skip it and you play with fate and your muscles and joints. This is a tough regimen, and in 10 days you will be healthy, slender and stronger in your fighting art, but only if you do it safely and intelligently.

Preparation

You have three weeks of prolonged effort ahead of you: careful eating, hard training, extra sleep, and not much else. First, check your calendar to see if any big events in your life fall within the 21 days. Is there a family reunion coming up, a week-long vacation or the Christmas holidays? If so, you might want to schedule your 21-day weight loss session so that it ends just before the event or it starts right after. By the way, if you begin the program after an event, don't rationalize that you can pork out at the festivities since you are going on a weight-loss program. Why would you want to put on three new pounds just before you begin suffering through three weeks trying to shed 10?

Enjoy the event, but control your eating and drinking.

The Right Mindset

Know that there is zero tolerance here for cheating, no matter how innocent. Keep in mind that that piece of candy you so desperately want would mean 30 minutes of training added to the additional training you are doing already. Or, to think of it another way, if you did an extra 30 minutes of bag work today and then later gave into that piece of candy, you just destroyed the calorie burning benefits of the bag work. Don't skip your workouts. A skipped workout will show up on your bathroom scale on the 21st day, as will all the times you failed to eat properly or get enough rest. Instead of 10 pounds, the scale might read only nine, or eight or . . . If you decide to accept an invitation to a party and eat lots of goodies and stay out so late that you can't possibly train the next day, the infraction will show up on your bathroom scale on the 21st day. Your priority right now is to train hard, eat right and get plenty of shuteye. Losing 10 pounds is tough, but it will happen if you follow the right path. Remember, it's all about the 21st day.

Some people find that it helps to place Post-it notes around their homes and in their cars as a not-so-subtle reminder to stay disciplined and to keep their eyes on the goal. Consider putting a rubber band on your wrist to snap painfully every time you are lured towards

"forbidden fruits." Put a before picture of yourself in a bathing suit on the refrigerator door as a reminder of why you are watching the calories and training so hard. Use whatever works so you don't cheat yourself out of getting the desired results.

Continually ask: Will doing this or eating that help me reach my goal? Or will it hurt me? Know that every step away from your goal necessitates that you take two additional steps in the right direction to make up for it. Two additional steps! Why make the task twice as hard as it already is? Stay on course with one eye on your calorie consumption and training regimen and the other eye on the calendar. Hey, there are people serving 21 years in prison. You just have to do this for 21 days. So cut the calories, do the work and in the end, when those 10 pounds are no longer part of you, feel good about yourself for a job well done. Strut a little and spend some time in front of the mirror.

Let's Get Physical

Before we hit you with the hard stuff, here is an easy and nifty training concept to use during the 21-day program, the 10-day program or any other time you want to use it.

One-Minute Training   Keep this simple fact in the forefront of your mind: Every time a calorie dies, you move that much closer to your goal. One-Minute Training is 60 seconds of sweatless fun that improves your technique while killing a dozen calories, give or take a couple. When you do a One-Minute session two, three, four or more times a day, in conjunction with your calorie cutting and the extra hard training sessions, the mini-workouts help keep your metabolism stoked like a red-hot furnace.

One-Minute Training can be done anywhere, at any time; all you need is 60 seconds. There is no need for a warm-up or to stretch since you aren't going all out. Decide on what you want to do and then concentrate on executing the movements with flawless form and a relaxed flow for one full minute. Do one while sitting in your car, sitting at your desk, while waiting for the coffee to percolate, during a television commercial, at the bus stop (though you may get some weird looks), in the bus (even weirder looks), in a cab, or in a restroom stall. The opportunities are endless; you just have to seize the moment, one 60-second moment to brutally murder a few extra calories and improve your martial arts skills a little.

Stir that imagination of yours to make your sessions interesting and beneficial. You can do something different each time and think of One-Minute Training only as a calorie burner, or you can do the same thing each time, and think of it as a calorie burner and a way to polish a specific technique. Here are a few other ideas:

• Imagine an opponent attacking you with different techniques as you block or parry each one. You can do them sitting at your desk, on your sofa, standing in your kitchen, leaning against a tree, or in an open space where you can practice footwork. If the urge comes over you while lying on the floor watching television, do 60 seconds of blocks as if defending against someone attacking while you are down. Do the same blocks every time, or free flow. Counter if you want.

• Pick one technique and work it for a minute. Does your backfist need extra work? Punch? Sidekick? Footwork? Evasive maneuvers? Hey, it's your minute: You choose. Strive for good technique and see if you can do 10 on your left side and 10 on your right before the 60 seconds are up.

• There is an old Chinese legend about a woman learning the martial arts in a style based on strong stances and powerful kicking techniques. To force her to concentrate on her legs, the teacher tied the woman's hands behind her back so that all day she had to use her feet for all that she usually did with her arms (hmmm, but how did she go to the...?) This unique training eventually turned this woman into an invincible kicker, so fast and so powerful that one day she used her great kicking skills to easily defeat a gang of marauding male bandits.

Though you don't need to actually bind yourself, you can still pretend you are a student of this master for 60 seconds. Stand before a closed door in your home, chamber your leg, extend it into a sidekick and open the door by the knob with your foot. Enter the room, chamber your other leg, execute a sidekick and close the door using the knob. Turn on the light switch with a right front kick and switch on the stereo with a left front kick. Let your creativity loose and experiment with whatever comes to mind (inserting a key into a lock is one of our favorites) for 60 seconds.

• Choose a troublesome form and do whichever section needs extra work for 60 seconds. You don't have to do low stances or aerial cartwheels, but rather use the time to work on technical perfection and a smooth flow. Besides burning a handful of calories, you benefit by imprinting the correct techniques into your memory so that they will be there when you practice the form in its entirety.

• Christensen talked about balloon kicking in *Solo Training: The martial arts guide to training alone*, and it can be a fun-filled one-minute exercise. Inflate a balloon with just enough air so that it stays airborne long enough to kick it, but not so full that it floats in the air for several seconds

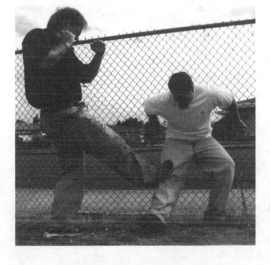

after. Strive for precise kicking, not speed and power, and use all your favorite kicks to keep the balloon from touching the floor for 60 seconds.

Use One-Minute Training throughout your day whenever you have a spare minute. Many fighters tell us that initially it's hard to remember to do the short sessions, but once they get into the groove, they find them addicting. One-Minute Training is a great way to stay in shape, engrain techniques, work out problems, burn a few calories, and burn off a little stress. If you want, you can even do Two-Minute Training sessions, though most people prefer just one minute.

Okay, let's kick the intensity up a notch and really start burning some calories to rid 10 pounds in 21 days.

Use big muscles   Punching and kicking are outstanding caloric burners, though one is more outstanding than the other. Your legs and buttocks are the largest muscle groups in your body and as such require more calories to move them through a kick than your relatively small arm muscles need to throw a punch. It makes sense, therefore, to do more kicking drills than punching drills during your 21-day quest for a leaner you. Here are five that will turn you into a lean, mean kicking machine, while burning calories at an accelerated rate:

Machine Gun Kicks

Perform the machine gun kicks explained in Chapter 8. Not only do they burn loads of calories, they increase your speed and develop knockout power.

Do 5 sets of 10 reps

Kicking Sets

Assume your fighting stance and execute two reps of any kick, say, front kick, before setting your leg back down into your fighting stance. Then execute three front kicks and again resume your fighting stance. Then four, and continue to add one in this manner until you have reached 10. Repeat with your other leg. To burn calories even faster, reverse the order. That means you execute 10 front kicks without stopping, and then return to your fighting stance. Then execute nine. Continue this countdown until you kick only one rep. Repeat with your other leg. One complete cycle is one set. Use your partner for a target, so that when you rest he performs a set, and vice versa.

Progressive set: Do two kicks on the first rep, and add a kick each rep until you do 10 kicks on the 10th rep.

Countdown reps: Do 10 kicks on the first rep, and do one less kick as you countdown to one kick.

Jump Kicks

Jump kicks require hard and fast muscle contractions to first propel your body airborne and then contract again to execute the kick. Begin in your fighting stance and execute 10 jumping front kicks with your right leg and 10 with your left. If you can do another type, say jump sidekick, do 10 of those with each leg. If you can kick simultaneously with both legs, do 10 beginning with your left side forward and 10 from your right side forward. The more jump kicks you can do, the more calories you burn from the double muscle contractions.

If you know only one jump kick: 3 sets of 10 reps, each leg.

If you know three types of jump kicks: 1 set of 10 reps of each kick, each leg

Warning: If you are 20 or more pounds over weight, it's recommended that you don't do jump kicks because of the added strain to your joints when landing.

Kneeling Kicking Drill

Stand before a heavy bag in your fighting stance, left leg forward. Lower your right knee until it almost touches the floor. To prevent lateral movement in your leg, which can injure your ligaments, your right heel points straight up as your right knee points straight down. Push your body forcefully into an upright position and drive a right front kick into the bag. Retract your kick and return it to the starting position with your heel up and your knee almost touching the floor.

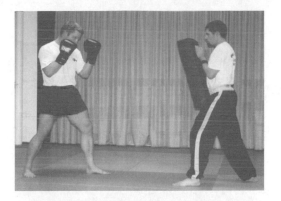

If this is new to you, start slowly until you get a feel for the movement. Once you are comfortable with it, go all-out. Since this drill leaves your leg muscles shaking and quivering like a newborn fawn's, it's best to do it only twice a week with at least two days in between.

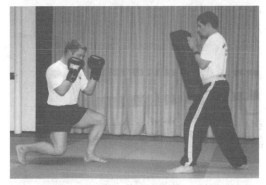

Front kick: 1 set of 10-20 reps, each leg

Roundhouse kick: 1 set of 10-20 reps, each leg

Sidekick: 1 set of 10-20 reps, each leg

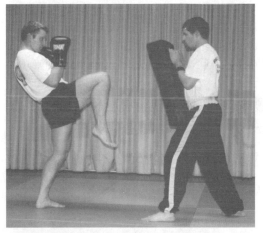

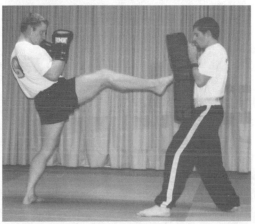

Mitt Kicking Drill

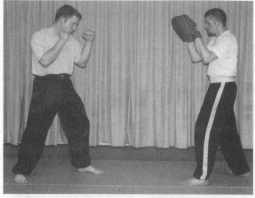

Assume a fighting stance and face a training partner holding a focus mitt on each hand at chest level. At his discretion, he jerks one arm behind him and either leaves the other mitt in front of his chest or moves it to another position. Your job is to respond instantly with a fast kick into the exposed mitt, in this case a hook kick. He then presents a mitt facing downward, which you front kick.

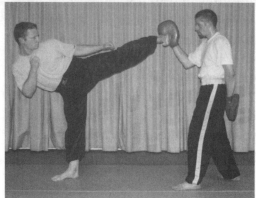

Your partner controls the tempo by how fast or slow he alternates the presentation of either the left or the right mitt. He uses footwork to force you into following him, as if you were pursuing a retreating opponent, though he should stay close enough so you can kick the mitts. This is a dynamic and challenging exercise, so begin slowly to get a feel for it and then increase the pace. If you start missing or hesitating too often, slow down. Switch roles with your partner after each round.

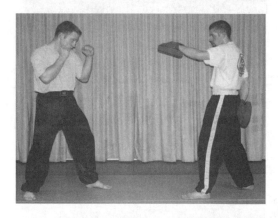

Do 3 one-minute round.

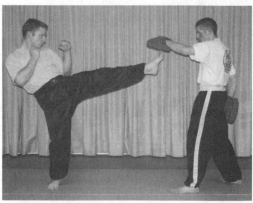

Sparring Sessions

Whether you practice the striking arts, grappling arts, or one that combines both, sparring is a demanding exercise that uses virtually every muscle in your body, especially your heart, as it thumps madly to carry oxygen and blood throughout your system. Unlike prearranged drills, you can't relax or get sloppy since your sparring partner will be all over you, chuckling like a happy demon. It's arguably the most challenging aspect of martial arts training, as it allows you to test your skills and try to outsmart your opponent. Your calorie-burning engine is revved to the max as you attack hard, fast and with versatility, while defending your opponent's continuous onslaught. Sparring is a wonderful calorie burning exercise that ultimately sharpens your fighting ability at the same time.

Here are a few ways to make it interesting:

- You don't have to go all-out every time to burn calories. Keep the pace at medium speed and focus on executing a variety of techniques. Choose a partner who also wants to experiment with lots of different moves, rather than just trying to beat you. Have fun and learn, but keep it non-stop to burn lots of calories.

Do 5, 5-minute bouts, with 2-minute rest periods in between

- Experiment with different parameters, such as speed, power, length of rounds, and length of rest periods. For example, throw your techniques fast but with only 75 percent power. This allows you to move as quickly as possible but with control. Then change the format to one in which you execute powerful techniques at medium speed. This is done by launching, say, a medium-speed reverse punch at your partner's chest, and then using the power of your hip rotation, the muscles of your arm and your abdominal muscles, push an inch or two deeper into the target. When using a kick, connect with your foot then use the muscles in your butt and legs to push it into the target an inch or two. Think of the action as pushing "through" the target.

Whether you are doing fast sparring with reduced power or power sparring with reduced speed, experiment with the length of the rounds and rest periods. For example:

2-minute rounds, 30 seconds rest
3-minute rounds, 60 seconds rest
4-minute rounds, 90-seconds rest

- Get your partner to put on as much padding as he can, while still able to move. The drill is to thump away on him non-stop for several rounds as he offers only minor resistance. Mostly, he is a walking heavy bag who blocks and attacks occasionally to keep you on your toes and prevent you from getting sloppy. In spite of the protective gear, your partner should expect to get banged up after a few rounds. Just remember that he gets to beat you up when it's his turn.

This is a great sparring exercise to help you learn to keep attacking as your energy and wind fades. When you switch roles, you learn to keep defending, though exhausted. It's a good idea to have a third party monitor and referee to ensure the defender is not getting too badly mangled in spite of the padding.

Do 3-5, 3-minute rounds with 60-second rest periods

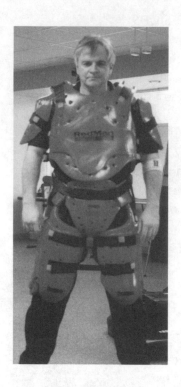

One-technique Fighters Burn Few Calories

Many fighters spar defensively, counterattacking only with single techniques, one punch or one kick. There are also offensive fighters who attack mostly with single techniques. While this might be exactly what the moment calls for, it's not conducive to burning many calories. If you are such a fighter, you need to force yourself, for the sake of burning fat during this 21-day period, to fight offensively and aggressively with multiple techniques. Who knows, you might like the new style.

Cycle Your Training to Avoid Overtraining

If any of the rapid calorie burning exercises in this chapter are more intense than you are used to, the new challenge will burn fat and help you progress in speed, strength, technique, power, and endurance. A word of caution: Inherent in these or any new training regimens is the potential to overtrain in intensity and duration, thus opening the door for Mr. Injury to come in. With calorie cuts and extra training, your body needs lots of rest to repair muscle tissue, strengthen tendons and bones, eliminate lactic acid, and simply restore your mental drive to do it again tomorrow. Should you fail to get your rest, your body has evil ways of letting you know that it doesn't like you any more. You feel physically drained, ill tempered and one part of your body hurts and another aches; you may even tear a tendon or break a bone. Training to exhaustion every day isn't beneficial in the long run, especially should you strain something and have to take two weeks or two months off to heal. Lying on the sofa and moaning does nothing for the waistline.

The solution is to cycle your major training sessions. If you enjoy an evening walk or you like to do two or three One-Minute Training sessions each day, continue to do them whenever you like, but your primary training sessions need to be cycled by using one of three levels of training intensity.

A-sessions These sessions are done at normal intensity. They are good, basic workouts that are neither grueling nor easy. You work up a sweat but you aren't left exhausted at the end of the session. A typical A-session would take 90 minutes, including your warm-up and cool-down. As a point of reference, consider the intensity of your regular classes to be A-sessions (if they were B- or C-sessions, it wouldn't be necessary for you to do this extra training). Any extra sessions done at home or during free time at your school should be done at level A.

B-sessions To make B harder than an A-session, you must increase the duration of your training by a few minutes, and the volume by 15 to 25 percent. So, if your normal session is 90 minutes, you want to add 15 to 30 minutes; never go past two hours. If you normally do 4 sets of 20 reps of any given exercise, you must increase to 5 sets of 25 reps.

C-sessions Hate us because we are more handsome than most, but don't hate us because we gave you the dreaded C-session. There is no holding back and no surrendering; you know it's over when you collapse into a fetal position. Okay, that is an exaggeration, but not by much. Maximum training time is 90 minutes, counting 15 minutes to warm-up and 15 to cool-down. In between are 60 super-intense training minutes.

Although the training duration goes down in C-sessions, the intensity shoots through the roof as each technique is executed at maximum speed and power. You want to sustain your heart rate around 80 percent of your maximum, or higher if you are in good shape. C-sessions are all about maximum intensity and maximum calorie consumption. It doesn't matter if you hit the heavy bag, spar, do your forms at full speed repeatedly, or shadowspar as if possessed. What does matter is that you go hard.

Determining Your Maximum Heart Rate

Here is how to determine your maximum heart rate and training heart rate. Although this is a relatively simplistic method and has received some criticism of late, it applicable to our needs here and has worked for athletes for many years.

Males, take the number 220 and females take the number 226 and subtract your age. The difference is your maximum heart rate. Multiply this by the percentage at which you want to train and the answer determines the heart rate you need to maintain throughout your aerobic session. We suggest you train at 80 percent unless you are terribly out of shape, in which case you should begin at about 60 percent and increase over the days as you see fit. (As always, get

your doctor's advice before beginning a rigorous program).

Here is how it looks if you are a 26-year-old female wanting to train at 80 percent of your maximum heart rate.

$226 - 26 = 200 \times .80 = 160$ beats a minute

Your pulse sites are on your wrists just above your thumbs and one on either side of your neck, about an inch below your ear on your jaw line. Stop your exercise and check one of the sites for six seconds and then immediately resume your activity. Multiply the number of beats you felt by 10. If you felt 16 beats, 16 multiplied by 10 is 160 beats per minute. If you are 26 years old female, you are right on target. If you counted 10 beats, you need to pick up the pace, but if you counted 20, you need to slow down, especially if you are feeling overtaxed.

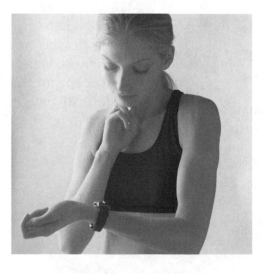

Tip: Don't skip or minimize your warm-up and cool-down periods for the sake of saving time. If your body isn't prepared for the intensity of a C-session, you have to make time for Mr. Injury.

Here is a simple schedule for cycling your sessions. Notice that the intensity increases gradually; so don't fret if you don't lose much weight the first few days. Think of the first week as preparation for the second and third one, a time to get in a few easy sessions so you can more easily adapt to the harder ones. Though you may feel fresh and eager after the first few days, don't yield to the temptation to train harder. Use the "easy" week wisely, as the next one is harder and the one after that is a killer.

Notice there is only one A-session the second week and lots of Bs and Cs, so expect to sweat. Your training is becoming more intense but still it's only a transition to the next level — the dreaded third week. Think of the last week as your own personal "Hell week" — remember the Navy SEALS? — when you get to test your warrior spirit and perseverance. Unlike the SEALS, however, you get to rest and eat well. Keep in mind as you groan through this third week that you are burning calories at an extraordinary rate. Hang in there as now your goal is within reach. Here is what your schedule looks like:

A Pep Talk

Hopefully, with all the tricks and tools you have been given for the task, losing five or 10 pounds of fat is less intimidating than you might have first thought. It's still a rough endeavor, but with knowledge, discipline and an iron will, success is just a matter of doing it. Just remember that there are no magic bullets, no matter how convincing the ads and infomercials may seem. The only bullet is the one you have to bite (some days you gnaw it) to get through the 10-day or 21-day plan. So, cue up the right mindset, eat healthily and train hard. A slimmer you is just a few days away.

Weeks	Mon	Tue	Wed	Thu	Fri	Sat	Sun
1	B	C	A	B	C	B	A
2	C	B	C	A	B	C	B
3	B	C	A	C	C	B	C

What if Things Don't Go As Planned?

Whenever you begin a weight loss plan with a specific end date, there is always the risk you won't achieve your goal, especially when the plan is for fast weigh loss. While some people have a naturally fast metabolism and lose weight easily, others have to fight for every ounce lost. Not only is your body incredibly complicated, but also your daily life doesn't always fit in well with your plans. There are parties, snack plates at work, an invitation for a beer with a buddy, and on and on. Even when you resist these temptations and do everything right, three or four days might pass before you see a drop on the scales. Or even worse, your weight loss on the final day might not be as large as you wanted. These are real possibilities and a primary drawback with quick weight loss plans that have an end date.

As we have said all along, there are no shortcuts to losing five or 10 pounds healthily. The methods we have given you are the best for the job, and have been proven to work in case after case. But, and this is a really big but, there are no guarantees. Losing excess weight quickly takes lots of effort: proper planning, preparation, increased training, regular eating patterns, reduced calories, and a sound healthy diet. Still, you are dealing with the human machine and sometimes it just has a will of its own.

However, there are a few things you can do when the scales are not going down as quickly as you had planned.

- Weigh yourself at set times, preferably in the morning after you have gone to the bathroom, before you eat breakfast and as naked as the day you came screaming into the world. This is the only way to be consistent in measuring your weight. People who weigh themselves in the evening after they have eaten several meals and consumed fluids all day won't get an accurate reading, since they weigh several pounds more than in the morning. Always weigh upon awakening in the A.M. to be sure you aren't worrying needlessly.

- Check your training schedule and be completely honest with your evaluation as to whether you might have strayed a little (or a lot) from your plan. Did you finish the 90 minutes session of all-out training or did you begin cooling down 10 minutes too soon? Did you work the heavy bag as hard as you could or were you holding back a little after the first set because your legs felt like lead? Be brutally honest with your evaluation. Only you can cheat yourself.

- Evaluate your diet. This is why it's so important to maintain a log of what you have eaten and how you have trained. If you don't like the logs in this book, use a little pocket notebook and carry it every minute of your day. Note everything you eat and drink. That means everything. No exceptions. If it goes into your mouth, write it down. Everything. (Have we made it clear that you need write down everything?) Refer to it often to calculate your calories and ratio of protein, carbs and fat. With an honest log, you can see where extra calories have snuck in and sabotaged your plan.

- Add an early morning, light cardio to your routine. Get out of bed, drink a glass of water and warm up slowly in preparation for a light workout. Go through your forms, shadow-box, rep drills, what-ever, just keep it light. Raise your heartbeat to, say 65 to 75 percent. Should you train at too high of an intensity, you might feel fatigued the rest of the day. A nice, light early morn-ing session not only helps you recover from your previous training day, it burns additional fat calories on an empty stomach.

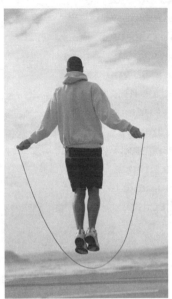

- Here is a neat little if-all-else-fails plan to trim that last, stubborn pound or two. Plan your 10 or 21 day train-ing so it ends on a weekend when there is a martial arts seminar, one that is physically challenging and gives you a good, all-day workout. Eat just enough for energy to get you through the sessions and don't go out with the others for a pizza after-wards. It's been a long 10 days or 21 days, so just go home and enjoy the fact that it's almost over. Tomorrow you might be sore and tired from the seminar, and drained from the grueling 10 or 21 day session, but feel

good that you have given it your best (but only if you have). Now shuffle over to the scale and be prepared for a fist pumping, "Yes!"

What Happens the Next Day?

Once it's over and you have shed five pounds (maybe four) on the five-pound diet, or 10 pounds (maybe nine) on the 10-pound diet, look at your notes and ponder all the hard work it took to get that feel-good number on the scales: training, discipline, self- control and all that you sacrificed and experienced during those 10 or 21 days. Now, burn those thoughts into your memory to motivate you to stay in shape and never again have to go through another quick-weight loss session.

Should you go back to your old ways that caused your weight gain, know that the pounds are going to come back with a flashing red light and a whaling siren. The solution? Don't go back to your old ways. To maintain your new weight, add 200 calories back into your daily diet and cut back a little on your training. If after a couple of weeks you are still losing, add another 100 calories and cut back a little more on your training. Continue in this fashion until your weight stabilizes where you want it. Now, if you have learned to like the hard training you did during the quick weight loss period and want to keep at it, good for you. Just add 200 calories a week until your weight stabilizes.

If in a few months you find that you are gaining again, say three or four pounds, don't feign surprise because you know exactly why it happened (yes, honesty hurts), but you also know how to get them off. Take immediate action so you never have to go through another 10- or 21-day plan. Tighten up your eating discipline and increase your training again until you shed those unwanted pounds. However, if you have slipped six, eight or 10 pounds and you have to shed it quickly, return to the beginning of this chapter.

Lose Sleep, Gain Weight

Sleep loss might increase hunger and affect your body's metabolism, which can make it more difficult to maintain or lose weight. CBS's The Early Show Medical Correspondent Dr. Emily Senay says better sleep habits might be the key to success of any weight management plan. She says studies have shown sleep loss affects the secretion of the appetite hormone cortisol. Sleep loss may also interfere with the body's ability to metabolize carbohydrates and cause high blood glucose levels. Excess glucose promotes the overproduction of insulin, which can promote the storage of body fat.

Fast Facts

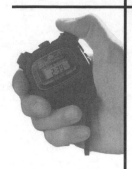

- It's been our experience teaching thousands of students for over 50 combined years that those who train with some kind of resistance exercises are better than those who don't.

- The more muscle you have, the greater your metabolic rate and the more calories you burn throughout the day.

- Your muscles are made up of three types of fibers, little motor units that contract when you punch and kick.

- You genetically inherited from your parents the ratio of fast-twitch and slow-twitch muscle fibers that you have right now.

- Your training objective for gaining additional muscle size isn't to pose on the beach, but to develop highly functional muscles that benefit your fighting.

- Long duration aerobics burns lots of calories and fatigues your muscles so you can't push as hard with dynamic tension or the weights.

- When your regular martial arts class includes lots of horse stance squats, one-legged squats, various forms of push-ups and dynamic tension, you will develop greater muscle size than a fighter who only practices kicking and punching.

- Dynamic tension has been an important supplemental exercise in the martial arts for many years.

- While there are many other weight resistance exercises, the three presented here target the largest number of muscles and those applicable to a host of martial arts movements.

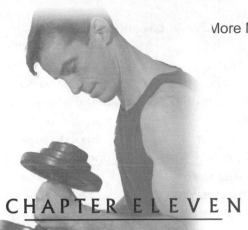

CHAPTER ELEVEN

More Muscle, More Power

Ever since Bruce Lee exploded onto the martial arts scene via television and the movies, our perception of martial arts fighting heroes and villains have been formed mostly by Hollywood and Hong Kong. Most are lean and muscular, and directors love to show their physiques in torn shirts, dramatic lighting and spray-on sweat. Rarely do we see overweight martial arts actors, Sammy Hung being the rare exception. Adding to our perception of the ideal fighting physique are today's full-contact fighters, many of whom rival bodybuilding contestants.

Lean, muscular physiques have been presented by the entertainment industry and in martial arts magazines for so long that many people — fans who don't train and people just beginning to — consider such musculature a standard in the fighting arts. Some even believe that ripped physiques can be developed by just practicing the martial arts. While that would be wonderful if it were indeed

the case, the reality is that we need to do more than just kick and punch. Yes, martial arts training when coupled with a proper diet often develops a lean physique with some degree of musculature, but to pack on extra muscular weight, one has to make an extra effort. Is it easy? Nope. Nothing worthwhile is.

Decades ago, weight training was considered in many martial arts circles to be detrimental to one's skill. There were absurd claims that larger than average muscles would slow a fighter down and interfere with ease of movement. While there is some truth to this when talking about a person in the top echelon of professional bodybuilding, few if any martial artists reach that caliber of muscularity, or want to.

It's been our experience teaching thousands of students for over 50 combined years that those who train with some kind of resistance exercises are better than those who don't. Can you be successful in your chosen fighting art without such training? Yes. Will you be better if you make resistance training part of your repertoire? Yes, at least in our experience and in the experience of many, many other instructors. We certainly don't believe that fighters need large and showy muscles, but when muscles are developed specifically to augment martial arts movements, their overall fighting improves dramatically.

In this section we look at ways to increase your bodyweight with muscle that is functional and applicable to your fighting art.

3 Ingredients to a Quality Weight Gain

There are three components to gaining healthy body weight:

- You must do specific free-hand exercises, dynamic tension or weight resistance exercises, the latter being the most beneficial for weight gain.

- You need a positive calorie balance, which means you take in more calories than you burn during your normal work or school day and in your martial arts training.

- You need lots of rest to allow your muscles to rebuild from the training.

Before providing you with solid tips on how to do this, let's take a quick look at the structure of your muscles and understand how it's possible for them to grow. Try not to nod off on us like you did in those biology classes in high school because having a basic understanding helps you progress.

Muscle Fibers

Your muscles are made up of muscle fibers, little motor units that contract when you punch and kick. There are three types:

Fast-twitch muscle fibers These are used when executing movements that are explosive, fast and powerful. A lightning-fast punch, a quick snap kick or an explosive takedown technique require that your muscles contract hard and fast. Although fast-twitch muscles contract nearly twice as fast as slow-twitch, they tire twice as fast, too.

Slow-twitch muscle fibers These are the exact opposite of fast-twitch. They are used for slow and repetitive movements, such as jogging or practicing your forms slowly and methodically. Slow-twitch muscles can work for a long time, far longer than fast-twitch.

Intermediate fibers Here you get the best of both worlds. Intermediate-twitch muscles work hard and fast and can do so for a long time. About 60 percent of people have predominantly intermediate muscle fibers. The remaining 40 percent are equally divided between slow and fast twitch.

Each person has a different ratio of muscle fiber types. Some have mainly fast-twitch muscle fibers, making them naturally gifted for fast and explosive movements. These people gravitate toward physical activities such as sprinting, long jumping and the martial arts. Some experts believe that Bruce Lee's extraordinary speed was a result of having predominately fast-twitch muscles. Other people have a predominant number of slow-twitch fibers, and they tend to gravitate towards endurance sports, such as long distance running or cycling. They can maintain a steady pace for hours, but they do poorly at short, fast sprints.

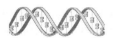

You Got Yours from Your Parents

You genetically inherited from your parents the ratio of fast-twitch and slow-twitch muscle fibers that you have right now. So if you got mostly slow-twitch muscles, there isn't anything you can do other than make the best of it (and never again call or write your parents). You can work around them, but it's beyond the scope of this book as to how that is done. Two books that address the issue are *Warrior Speed* by Ted Weimann, published by Turtle Press and *Speed Training* by Loren Christensen, available at www.lwcbooks.com.

While slow-twitch and intermediate twitch are capable of growing larger, it's the fast-twitch ones that respond better to strength developing exercise. But this doesn't mean you should only do exercises that activate your fast-twitch muscles. It's more productive to train all three groups of muscle fibers.

Resistance Exercises

Your training objective for gaining additional muscle size as a martial artist isn't to pose on the beach, but to develop highly functional muscles that benefit your fighting techniques. However, a happy byproduct of your training is that you will gain some appreciable muscle size. The single most effective way to gain size and body weight is through progressive resistance exercises: free-hand exercises, dynamic tension training and weight training. Now, if you hate these types of exercises, sorry, but there is no way around it. To gain practical size and power for hard hits and dynamic throws, you have to make friends with barbells and dumbbells, weight machines, dynamic tension and free-hand exercises that allow you to increase resistance as you grow progressively stronger.

Free-hand Exercises

Free-hand exercises, such as push-ups, sit-ups, squat jumps, jumping jacks (side straddle hops) are great exercises but not conducive to adding much bodyweight. Now, if you are terribly out of condition and haven't been following any type of exercise program, you just might add muscle mass from free-hand exercise as long as you eat properly and get sufficient rest. Soldiers in boot camp frequently gain weight from such exercises.

Kick boxer and author of *Fighting Science*, Martina Sprague, uses free-hand exercise along with weight training and jogging. "For upper body strength, I recommend push-ups, dips and pull-ups. For lower body strength, I recommend running on hills and squat jumps. I average 50, full-range push-ups, 10 pull-ups and 250 to 300 sit-ups of some variety every day. I definitely believe in weight resistance and other forms of resistance training. I have found that the simplest training methods to be best."   So have we.

Don't Overdo the Aerobics

Review your aerobic training to see if you might be doing too much. Long duration aerobics burns lots of calories and fatigues your muscles so you can't push as hard with dynamic tension or the weights. In extreme cases, aerobics actually waste away your hard-trained muscles. Your goal and focus right now is to increase your muscular development, not improve your aerobic condition. If you insist on doing them, limit the sessions to 30 minutes, three times a week. You can always do more once you finish building the muscle you want. More on this later.

Kick-punch Arts

By saying that resistance training is the most effective way to gain muscle size and power doesn't imply that martial arts training is ineffective. Actually, there are three ways you can gain muscle using the fighting arts, each greater than the last.

• Most striking arts use explosive, powerful movements in training that stimulates the fast-twitch muscles in large and small muscle groups. If that is all that you do, meaning that you don't do additional supplemental exercises, you will develop a lean, hard physique — as long as you follow a good diet.

• When your regular martial arts class includes lots of conditioning exercises, such as horse stance squats, one-legged squats, various forms of push-ups and dynamic tension, you will develop greater muscle size than a fighter who only practices kicking and punching. Of course, you must eat correctly, too.

• When you supplement your martial arts training with resistance training of some kind — free weights, machines and dynamic tension — you get the greatest muscle growth, as long as you eat and sleep correctly.

Grappling Arts

There is a component of resistance to most grappling arts (judo and jujitsu, but very little in aikido) by virtue of how they are practiced. You push and pull as hard as you can against an opponent who pushes and pulls as hard as he can, all of which involve fast-twitch muscles. This is a form of resistance exercise, especially when you and your opponent are evenly matched strength wise. Grappling provides some muscle development, more than in the striking arts but not as much as weight training. Except for genetically gifted people (those who gain muscle easily), you won't develop large, bulging muscles from participating in the grappling arts. The good news is the size and strength you do gain is directly applicable to your fighting art.

It's important to reiterate that neither this chapter nor this book is about developing showy muscle. There are hundreds of books on the subject, magazines, videos, and internet sites. Our purpose here is to give you some ideas as to how to use nutrition, the martial arts and supplemental exercise to add size and power to your punching, kicking and throwing muscles.

Let's take a quick look at exercises that increases your strength and, when combined with a proper eating plan we discuss in a moment, pack on quality weight.

Dynamic Tension

Dynamic tension is a simple, but highly effective way for your muscles to gain power and increase size by working against other muscles in your body. You control the tension by increasing or decreasing the amount of resistance you apply. The exercises are considered progressive because you continuously increase the tension as you progress in strength.

Dynamic tension has been an important supplemental exercise in the martial arts for many years. It defines the word applicability because it develops power from the starting point of a technique and all along its track. This is called "specificity of movement," meaning that you exercise the exact muscles you want to increase in power and size.

Advantages   You can do dynamic tension as a supplement along with your weight training, by itself at the end of your martial arts workout, or on those days you don't train in your fighting art. If you normally lift weights but for whatever reason you can't for a while, dynamic tension helps maintain your weight-trained gains.

How it works   Any time you move your arm or leg, your muscles contract to a lesser or greater degree depending on what it is you are doing. For example, say you bend your right arm to touch your shoulder with your hand. Even when your hand is empty, the muscle fibers in your biceps shorten and contract to overcome gravity, though few are involved since your arm isn't terribly heavy and gravity isn't pulling it downward to any great degree.

Since not many fibers are activated — meaning you are using only a small portion of your available strength — all the other fibers are stretched out on little lawn chairs feeling smug at how easy they got it. To get those lazy ones off their bu-, uh, lawn chairs, especially the fast-twitch fibers, you have to pick up a heavy dumbbell and curl it to your shoulder. If there isn't a dumbbell available, you can activate roughly the same number of fibers by using your other hand to provide resistance to the curling motion.

Warm-up   Never skip the warm-up. We have seen and experienced many avoidable injuries when this all-important phase has been skipped. A cold muscle can get hurt just as easily doing dynamic tension exercises as it can doing a high kick or a heavy bench press when cold. Lots of fighters do dynamic tension near the end of their martial arts training session to take advantage of their already warm muscles, and this is fine. However, if you choose to do them on those days you don't practice martial arts, be sure to warm-up for at least 10 minutes. It gets real ugly when you actually hear a cold muscle snap (if you hear a twanging sound and you aren't playing

a guitar, you are in deep trouble). Speaking of injuries, it's important to use good form in every movement. Doing them wrong - which can happen easily when you are contracting so hard — imprints bad technique and puts the muscle at risk of making that twanging sound. Focus on maintaining perfect form.

There are lots of dynamic tension exercises and once you get familiar with them, you can even make up a few specific to your needs. If you want to explore the subject further, we suggest you check out Harry Wong's book *Dynamic Tension* published by Unique Publications. It's a wonderful guide that contains a variety of dynamic tension exercises applicable to the martial arts. Here are three basic ones to get an idea of what they feel like and how they apply to your martial arts:

Straight Punch

Begin by assuming a medium-low horse stance, a position from which you can practice a host of dynamic tension punches and blocks. Let's do a straight punch. Extend your left hand and chamber your right where you do normally. Christensen favors a high guard like a boxer, so he is shown chambering high, as opposed to chambering at the hip. As you s-l-o-w-l-y begin to pull back your left hand, punch s-l-o-w-l-y with your right, while contracting the muscles in your arms, abs, chest, and back as hard as you can. Apply as much tension to your retracting left arm as you do to your right. Do both s-l-o-w-l-y and with eye-popping intensity. Imagine there are mighty forces resisting your fists, making them move ever so slowly and your arms tremble from the exertion. When your right arm reaches full extension, relax for two seconds and then begin to slowly punch with your left and slowly retract your right.

Do 2 sets of 10 reps per arm

Many hand techniques can be executed while using your free hand to provide resistance.

Straight Punch with Resistance

Assume the same stance as just described. Position your left hand in front of your abdomen and block it with your right palm. Resist hard with your right as you push vigorously through the track of your left punch. Contract the muscles in your abs, chest, shoulder, arms and wrist as you push. Retract your left to the starting position and repeat.

Do two sets of 10 reps per arm

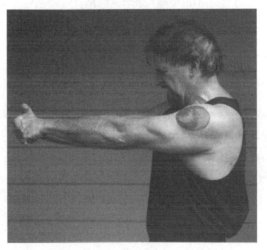

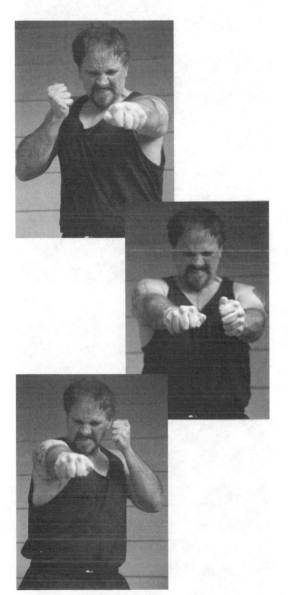

You can do the backfist motion without resistance, following the same procedure as you did in "Straight punch" or you can do it while resisting with your opposite hand. Here is how to do it with resistance:

Backfist with Resistance

Assume your fighting stance, left side forward. Wrap your right hand around your left fist and resist with your right as you begin to slowly move your left fist through the track of a head-high backfist. Contract the muscles in your abs, chest, shoulder, arms and wrist as you push against your right hand that provides enough resistance so that all your backfisting muscles are straining and trembling from the effort. When your backfist has reached full extension, move your right hand around to the palm side of your left fist to provide resistance for the retraction phase of the technique.

2 sets of 10 reps

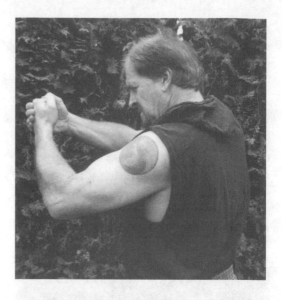

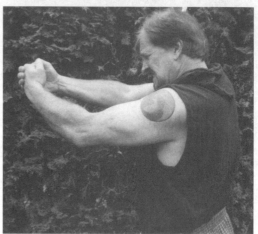

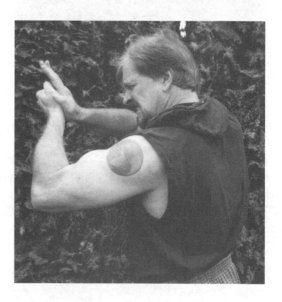

Kicks

You can use your normal on-guard position to perform most of your kicks with dynamic tension. It doesn't matter what kick you do as long as you do it slowly and with maximum tension. Since there is a tendency to speed up when losing your balance, hold on to something with one hand so all your concentration goes into maximizing your slow muscle contraction, which includes the muscles in your chest, abs, buttocks, thighs, and calves. While your primary emphasis is the kicking leg, contract the muscles in your support leg, too. Should you experience cramping in the hamstrings, upper thighs and butt, stop for a few seconds to let it subside or take a moment to shake it out. Cramping often occurs with extreme contraction, but it can also be caused by poor warm-up prior to exercising. Never skip the warm-up.

Do 2 sets of 10 reps per leg for each kick performed

Alternating full speed with dynamic tension   An interesting and taxing variation is to mix full-speed techniques with dynamic tension. This allows you to work those fast-twitch muscles two ways: First, do one rep of a punch or kick at maximum speed and power, then follow immediately with one rep using dynamic tension. Taxing? You bet, but power and size will be yours for the effort. Here is how it's done using a reverse punch.

Reverse punch: Begin by standing before a heavy bag in your on-guard position and throw a right reverse punch as hard and fast as you can into the vinyl or canvas. That is one rep. The second rep is done with dynamic tension, either by resisting with your free hand, or by punching without resistance but with maximum, arm shaking tension. After completing that rep, immediately drive a lightening fast punch into the bag. Keep alternating until you have completed a set of 10 reps with your right punch, a total of five fast and five with dynamic tension. Repeat with your left hand. Do this using as many different hand techniques or kicks as you want or have energy to do.

Do 2 sets of 10 reps per technique, per hand.

Dynamic tension is tough but it's highly effective for building strength and explosiveness in the exact movements in which you want to be strong and explosive. Coupled with correct eating (discussed in a moment), these exercises add a measure of muscle size and body weight to your physique.

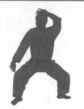

Fighting Styles that Practice Dynamic Tension

Some fighting styles, such as Isshin ryu, Shito-ryu, Hung gar, Goju-ryu and Uechi-ryu, focus heavily on dynamic tension, not only in their strength building exercises but also in their forms, which they combine with powerful breathing techniques. In some schools the teachers whack their students with sticks to test for muscle tension and mental focus.

If this is of interest to you, you might want to find a teacher in one of these styles and ask if he teaches dynamic tension as part of the curriculum. You can either join the school or just attend a few classes to learn how to apply it to your kata and other exercises you do.

Resistance Training and Old Fashioned Exercises

Many fighting systems use strength-developing exercises that have been passed down from old masters. Many of them are excellent for gaining martial arts power and additional muscle size, but at the risk of offending some teachers, many old exercises still being used today are potentially dangerous to the shoulders, lower back and leg muscles, and to the joints, ligaments and tendons in the fingers, wrists, elbows, ankles, and knees.

For example, the "duck walk," where one squats as low as possible and then walks, is a knee injury waiting to happen. Similarly, squatting with a fellow student on the shoulders is risky to everything from the lower back to the toes, since the rider can suddenly shift his weight or simply weigh more than the squatter can safely handle. Though push-ups on the fingertips are done in many schools, it's risky because it often causes tendon injuries, necessitating a trip to an orthopedic doctor.

A little knowledge can save you a lot of grimacing. Along with your study of the fighting arts, it's incumbent on you to learn about safe and dangerous exercises. Proper exercise will pack quality pounds on your body, but unsafe exercises just might cause you problems the rest of your life. Many of co-author Christensen's old injuries are a testament to bad exercises and old fashioned training procedures in his early years. We are certainly not saying that all traditional exercises are bad, nor are we saying that all modern exercises are safe. We are saying that it's important in your study to learn what is and isn't dangerous to you.

3 Exercises that Increase Power and Body Weight

Let's look at three weight exercises that will pack on muscle that is directly applicable to your fighting power and speed. To reiterate, we aren't talking about the showy kind, but rather muscle that is functional. Yes, a nice biceps muscle looks impressive in your bathroom mirror, but it's not going to do you a heck of a lot of good when Brutus the Bruiser is doing a Picasso with your facial features. More than bulging biceps, you want a punch that can penetrate oak doors and a kick that can dent an armor truck. The following exercises help you reach that objective, while adding some quality pounds, too.

Bench Press

There is a minor debate in bodybuilding circles as to whether the bench press is a good chest exercise. Well, we don't care about the argument because we use it to strengthen the shoulders, triceps, back and chest, the major muscles pertinent to punching, backfisting and pushing in the grappling arts. Applicability to punching is easily accomplished by precise placement of your hands on the bar.

Lie on a horizontal bench and place your feet flat on the floor or put them on the bench for added support. It doesn't matter as long as you are stable. Your head, shoulders and buttocks should remain on the bench at all times, though a slight arch in your back is okay: keyword, slight. For bodybuilding purposes, hand placement for the bench press is typically wider than the shoulders, but to replicate the punch, grab the bar with a grip shoulder-width apart and lift it off the rack. Inhale as you lower the bar at a controlled rate until it almost touches your chest and then drive it up to the starting position. Exhale as you pass the most difficult part of the press, the so-called "sticking point."

3 to 4 sets, 8 to 12 reps

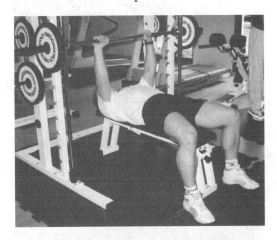

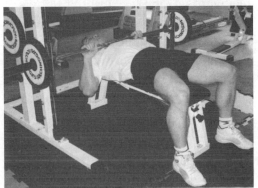

Some fighters prefer to use dumbbells because the motion feels more like executing a punch. If you prefer them, simply follow the same procedure as with the bar

3 to 4 sets, 8 to 12 reps

The weight should be sufficient to make you strain a little on the ninth and tenth rep. There is no need to pack so many plates on the bar that your blood vessels pop out and you have to kick and writhe on the bench to get up those last reps. You aren't trying to set a record here, but working to develop strong muscles that increase the power of your martial arts techniques.

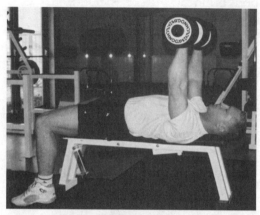

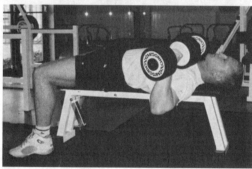

Bench press tips   Be careful not to arch too much, which allows the bar to move sideways, forwards or backwards. Don't lock out the elbows at the top of the press and don't bounce the weight off your chest. Your elbows don't have to rub your sides, but don't let them swing out too far, either. Remember, you are mimicking the punch. In fact, mentally "punch" the weight upward, thinking of each rep as a simultaneous double punch you are driving upward and into the target.

Squat

The squat exercise in its many forms has been around forever because it works. It builds power, explosiveness and muscular size. As a martial arts exercise, it develops power in all the kicks, particularly the front and roundhouse, and it develops strength and stability in your stances. There is really nothing bad to say about squatting except that when you do it hard you walk funny afterwards.

Stand up straight under the bar with your feet shoulder width apart and slightly turned outward. Hold the barbell behind your head, gripping it with a slightly wider than shoulder-width grip, and let it rest on your shoulders. Inhale and hold your breath as you begin to squat, allowing your upper body to lean forward a little (without changing the natural arch of your spine). Stop when your thighs are parallel to the ground, or sooner, depending on your strength and flexibility. Push yourself back up towards the starting position and exhale when you pass the sticking point. Think of the upward thrust as if driving a front kick through a heavy bag.

3 to 4 sets, 8 to 12 reps

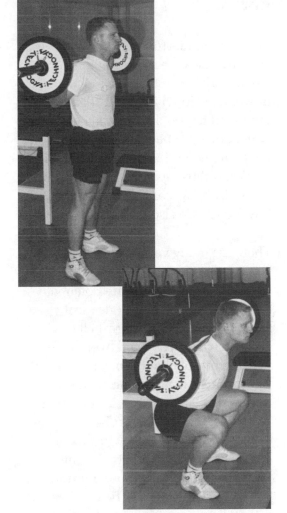

Squatting tips   Do be cognizant to keep your spine in a normal arch and that your knees travel over your feet, not to the outside or inside. Don't lock your knees at the top of the squat, rest at the top, lift your heels, or bounce at the bottom of the squat.

You can also squat while holding dumbbells, which doubles to strengthen your grip. If you have access to a Smith machine, leg press machine or hack squat machine, they too work well and offer a greater degree of safety than do free weights.

Rowing

This is a wonderful exercise that approximates the motion of the punch, particularly the retraction and all movements in which you pull an opponent to you. Rowing hits your large, powerful back muscles, especially the large, wing-like Latissimus dorsi (lats) and those surrounding your spine. Your biceps, forearms, shoulders and lower back are also worked.

There are many variations on the rowing exercise, most of which are excellent, though some are potentially dangerous. Perhaps the one most hazardous is the classic barbell rowing exercise where you bend over at the waist, grasp the handle of a barbell, lift it to your chest, and return it to the floor. There are many weight trainees who wish they had never heard of this exercise, especially in the morning when they awaken and their aching lower back snickers, "Good morning. Do you like the pain?" The good news is that there are weight machines today that mimic this movement but don't stress the lower back. They are definitely worth checking out.

Dumbbells are easier to manipulate, and they duplicate the actions of retracting a punch or pulling someone into you. Here is how you should do them.

Place your left knee on a horizontal bench with your ankle extending over the end. Place your left arm on the bench for support, so that your upper body is parallel to the ground while maintaining a normal arch to your back. Position your right leg a comfortable distance from the bench and put the majority of your weight on your left hand and leg. You should feel comfortable and stable.

Grip the dumbbell so your palm faces your body, inhale and hold your breath as you lift the weight as high as you can, at least above the level of your back. Once your elbow is at its highest point, raise the shoulder of the working arm to get an extra contraction in your back muscles. Exhale as you slowly lower the dumbbell back to the starting position. 3 to 4 sets, 8 to 12 reps

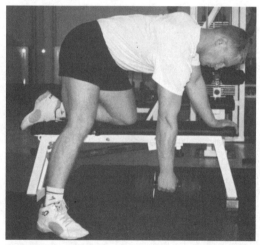

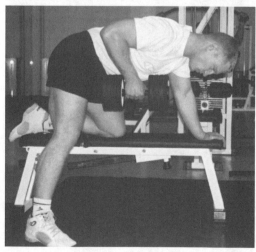

Rowing tips   Typical errors are failure to keep a normal arch in the back, rotating the torso, jerking the weight, curling the arm so the biceps does the work, and pushing off with the support leg.

Some people find it difficult to align the back correctly when using the knee and arm support method. Here is a good variation. Keep both feet on the floor and support your upperbody with only your hand on the bench. This prevents your back muscles from relaxing too much by forcing them to contract harder in order to maintain correct alignment in your spine.

While there are many other weight resistance exercises, the three presented here target the largest number of muscles and those applicable to a host of martial arts movements. When coupled with the right diet and plenty of sleep, muscle power, size and an increase in body weight are yours. Now let's check out what you have to eat.

Eat to Gain Weight Without Feeling Sluggish

Consider what a painfully skinny student once told co-author Christensen: "I drink a six-pack of beer a day just to keep some weight on my body. If I don't drink the beers, I drop pounds and get even skinnier." While his solution does sound intriguing (especially if you get a bag of chips, too), consuming empty calories and risking alcoholism isn't the answer. You want to gain weight from high quality, nutritious food that yields lots of energy while increasing lean muscle tissue. The tricky part is to eat in such a way that you gain muscle, not fat, and you feel comfortable, rather than sluggish from the extra calories.

Calories and Protein

Just as our approach to calorie reduction for weight loss is conservative, we favor a conservative approach to weight gain through a gradual and systematic increase in calorie consumption. Dynamic tension and weight training exercises fatigue your body by "damaging" or "tearing down" your muscles. To rebuild them with just a little more muscle and a little more strength after each workout, you need to rest, relax, get quality sleep, and feed your muscles good protein, the building blocks of a strong, muscular body.

The big question, one that is always controversial, is how much protein do you need? As discussed in previous chapters, there are protein diets out there that are so extreme that they dangerously overload your kidneys from the stress and strain of trying to assimilate the excessive grams. This is unnecessary. While you do need extra protein, you need to proceed conservatively. Begin by increasing your intake with 200 to 300 extra calories of protein each day. Please note that we said calories, not grams of protein; there is a huge difference.

One eight-ounce glass of skim milk supplies nine grams of protein, no fat, and 90 calories. Knock back three extra glasses a day and you get 27 grams of protein at 270 calories. A can of tuna packed in water contains 175 calories, 25 grams of fat and 37 grams of protein. Add a glass of skim milk and you get 90 more calories for a total of 265 and nine more grams of protein for a total of 46 extra grams of protein for the day. When you approach weight gain conservatively, you won't overwhelm your digestive system with lots of extra heavy food, you won't overload your kidneys with protein and you won't feel like a slug during your workouts.

Protein powders   Arguably the best way to increase your protein intake is with a good, fat-free whey protein supplement. Choose one that dissolves easily in water or skim milk, as opposed to the kind that needs to be mixed in a blender, and drink two to three servings a day. Since the calorie count is listed on the label, you know exactly how many you are getting, which helps to track your progress. The protein powder we use has 150 calories per scoop, 16 grams of whey protein, no fat, no cholesterol, and is fortified with vitamins. With powders, you also know you are getting a good quality protein, as opposed to a calorie-dense, fat-ribboned steak that tastes great but can cause bloat and leave you moving like a rhino.

Nutrition bars   There is nothing like finishing a hard workout and reaching into your gym bag to retrieve a low-cal (some as low as 150 calories), chocolate-covered nutrition bar packed with 20 grams of protein. If you choose well, it's all good protein that goes straight to your exhausted and needy muscles. In less than two minutes of chewing pleasure (though some brands taste like dog food), you satisfy your hungry body's need for muscle repair and building, and your taste bud's craving for sweets.

Supplement Means Supplement

Supplements are easy and quick way to get a shot of protein: Just dump a scoop of powder in a glass, or tear the wrapper off a bar. However, keep in mind the function of a supplement, which is to complement your regular food. Don't replace all your meals with them, but use them in addition to your regular meals when you need a quick 200 to 300 extra calories of muscle building protein. It's vital to eat as many nutritious meals as your busy life allows since they contain lots of important micronutrients not found in shakes and bars.

The Dark Side of Bars and Shakes

- **Too many calories** The old sage says, "Everything in moderation," and if he were expounding on supplements he would tell us to tread softly with bars and shakes. Since they are so easy to use and so perfect for your 100-mph lifestyle, they can easily become addictive, so much so that you might inadvertently take in more calories than you need. Many people have found that although they initially used bars and protein shakes for their convenience, they soon began using them as a comfort food, something to satisfy their craving for a treat. Though loaded with nutrition, bars and protein shakes still contain calories. As we say so often in this book that it will soon become a mantra, it's all about calories. Take in more than you need, even when deliberately trying to gain weight, and you get fat.

- **Not a complete meal** No matter how crammed the nutrition data appears on the labels, protein shakes and nutrition bars still don't provide all the nutrients you need each day. Your punching and kicking body also needs vegetables, meat and carbs from regular sources that contain the all-important micronutrients (certain minerals and vitamins) often missing in supplements. Is it possible to live exclusively on supplements? Probably. Can you do it healthily? No, because something on your person will eventually break, stop working or wither away. To avoid this annoy- ance, eat at least two well-rounded meals a day and use the supplements to, well, supplement.

- **Hard on the cash flow** Supplements tend to be expensive. If you get addicted to them, you could end up paying a couple of hundred dollars a month, or more. Even if this amount weren't a problem for your budget, it would indicate that you are abusing them and taking in too many calories, not getting enough nutrition, or both. If you are on a tight budget, it's worth the effort to eat regular food and prepare healthy lunches, mid-morning and mid-afternoon snacks to carry with you throughout the day. Use bars and shakes only when you are on a time crunch or need an extra hit of protein, say two or three times a week.

- **Some taste like *#%!!** Not all bars and shakes have a pleasant taste (and that is putting it nicely). Sometimes you have to test a lot of bars and drinks before you find one you can tolerate. Sometimes you just have to settle for one that is bearable and hope you get used to it. Know ahead of time that none of them tastes as good as pie alamode.

- **Not a magic bullet** By themselves, bars and shakes won't accelerate your progress in the martial arts, pack on muscle, strip off fat, or turn your wimpy sidekick into one that sends the biggest and toughest opponent rolling across the floor. They are simply supplemental food, nothing more.

The Bright Side of Bars and Shakes

- **Easy to find** Most grocery stores chains now carry nutrition bars in their health section, candy section or near the cash register.

- **Stick a bar in your pocket** Most bars are of a convenient size so you can hide one in your pocket at work or school, and chomp it down in two big bites.

- **Premixed shakes** There are companies that offer premixed formulas. All you do is pop the lid and take a swig.

- **Easy to digest** Keep looking until you find a product you enjoy for flavor and compatibility with your digestive system.

- **Helps to keep your energy up and level** Many of our students who lead busy schedules in school or in the work place use these supplements to keep their energy levels continuously up when a regular lunch or coffee break isn't possible.

- **Calorie, carb, fat and protein count made easy** One big advantage supplements have over your bologna sandwich is that they have labels that detail the products' nutritional information. Since some companies tend to exaggerate the term "healthy," check the fat and sugar content before you buy.

Monitoring Your Weight Gain Progress

First, be sure to get enough extra protein each day. As mentioned, begin your program by adding about 200 to 300 extra calories worth of protein to your diet, and at least 100 calories worth immediately after your training. A 10-ounce glass of skim milk provides around 100 calories and 10 grams of protein. If you supplement with one scoop of whey protein powder each day, drink the 16 grams of protein and 150 calories after your workout. Get your other 50 or 150 calories of protein at some other time during the day.

Next, keep good track of your weight gain by investing in a small body composition-measuring device, or go to a health club and ask to use theirs. With calipers or any of the more superior fat measuring devices mentioned in Chapter 3, you can determine immediately if you need to increase or decrease your extra protein calories. Let's say that when you begin your weight gain program you weigh 200 pounds with 15 percent body fat. After a month of hard training and protein supplementation, you show one of the following results.

- If your body fat still measures 15 percent but you now weigh 201 pounds, feel good about having added one pound of muscle. Don't change a thing you are doing.

- If you dropped to 14 percent body fat, and you still weigh 200 pounds, you trimmed fat but didn't gain muscle. Either your resistance training isn't hard enough or you didn't get enough protein, or both. You need to make adjustments.

- If you dropped to 14 percent body fat and added a pound of body weight, bringing you to 201, you lost fat and packed on lean muscle. You are training hard and eating right, so don't change anything.

When There are Problems

There are no bells or whistles to this approach, just a basic, proven method for gaining lean muscle mass. In a nutshell: Work out hard and add a little protein to your diet. That said, we don't want to oversimplify this process, as there are many factors that can cause problems to gaining muscle and adding bodyweight. So here is what we suggest.

For a couple of weeks before you begin this program, use your training log to jot down your workout regimen, diet, the hours you sleep, work habits on the job, and your school activities. If your routine remains the same after you begin your weight gain program, the added resistance exercises and extra protein should provide you with

weight and muscle gains in 30 to 60 days. However, if you don't see any improvement at all, you need to add a little more dynamic tension or weight training, and increase your daily protein intake another 150 to 200 calories (roughly 15 to 20 grams of protein).

When you examine your training log after a couple of months, it's important to be completely honest. Were you consistent in doing all the muscle-building sessions for which you were scheduled? If you missed a few, how many? Two? Ten? Are you doing too much cardio? Are you getting enough sleep? Remember, those late hours play havoc on your recuperation. If you have been keeping a detailed and accurate training log, the answer to your problem most likely will be on those pages.

Maybe you are successful after all
Before you get suicidal know that you just might be making gains. If you have been training hard and eating right, you might have lost a pound or two of fat and gained a pound or two of muscle. Since your bathroom scale doesn't know the difference, it will show the same weight 60 days later that you started with. A body composition caliper device, however, reveals the truth, and thus stops you from deliberately falling on your bayonet.

It's a feel-good plan What our students like about this conservative eating plan is that it doesn't leave them feeling sluggish and over-stuffed, so they have lots of energy and motivation to train. Many people err by taking the wrong path to weight gain by pigging out on too many carbs, fat grams and an excessive amount of protein, believing that more is better to pack on size. Yes, you do need more calories in your diet as your muscle size increases, but within reason. Take in too many, and your love handles grow right along with your biceps. However, when adding only a moderate 200 to 300 additional calories of protein, you eliminate the chance of overeating carbs and fat.

When you get your weight to where you want it, use your training log to determine how many calories you need to maintain your new, lean body weight. You might have to adjust down 200 or more, or increase up 200 or more until you get it right.

Creatine

Although there is some weight gain from water retention, creatine isn't a gain-weight supplement in the strictest sense of the term. However, it has an indirect positive effect on your weight gain progress because it helps your muscles contract better than without it. The harder they contract, the more muscle fibers you use and the more power you apply to your dynamic tension and weigh training exercises, all of which increases their size and strength.

Creatine is 100 percent natural and has been in our bodies since Adam and Eve, but it wasn't until the mid-1990s that everyone pumping weights and others training in various athletic activities began talking about its virtues and how best to use it as a supplement.

An Unscientific Experiment

Around 1996, co-author Christensen decided to give creatine a try, though he was a little dubious since as he had tried just about everything during his less than illustrious bodybuilding career 15 years earlier. He bought a big container, did the loading phase of taking in several scoops of the stuff for five days in a row, and then followed with two scoops daily for the next several months.

To determine if there was an improvement in his strength, he chose to experiment with just one exercise: barbell shrugs on a Universal bench press machine, one of the stations on the multi-station apparatus. With the bench scooted out of the way, he could grasp the bench press handles and perform shrugs to work his trapezes, that thick sheath of muscle that runs along the top of the shoulders and blends into the neck. To perform the exercise, he gripped the handles at arm's length along his thighs, lifted his shoulders to his ears, and then lowered his shoulders. The motion looks like the exerciser is doing reps of the nonverbal "I-don't-know." Teenagers are great at this exercise.

Christensen began the experiment with 80 pounds, a weight he could do easily for three sets of 10 reps. He could have lifted more, but he wanted the weight to be one that he could perform without any grunting or body cheating.

For the next three months, he maintained a daily creatine intake of 10 grams mixed in water. He performed the shrugs twice a week, adding weight when he could do so comfortably, usually once every two weeks, sometimes once a week. Again, the plan was to lift the poundage without struggle. His diet went unchanged for the test period, and he didn't do anything differently with the rest of his lifting routine or his martial arts training.

Three months later, he performed - drum roll, please — three sets of 10 fairly easy reps with 240 pounds. He said he could have lifted more but felt that some of the surrounding muscles that hadn't been strengthened along with his trapezes, might have given out with a big *riiiip!*

In no way should Christensen's study be labeled scientific. But as a guy who has experimented with all kinds of supplements over the years, he felt that creatine lived up to its press.

What Is It?

Your liver naturally combines three amino acids — arginine, clycine and methionine - to make creatine, and you also get it from the food you eat, such as herring, salmon, tuna, beef, and in supplement form. Once your liver transports creatine to your body's muscles through your bloodstream, it's converted into phosphocreatine (creatine phosphate), a high-powered metabolite used to regenerate your muscles' ultimate energy source, ATP, adenosine triphosphate (try saying that when eating taffy). It's believed that 95 to 98 percent of the creatine in your body is stored in your muscles, with the remaining two to five percent stored in various other places, including your brain, heart and testes.

Consider the internal workings of your sidekick. As you step, chamber and thrust, stores of energy (that ATP stuff) break down to give your leg the zip needed to make a big *whump!* on the heavy bag. When your leg retracts, your phosphocreatine stores are now mildly drained but your body works quickly to resynthesize (rebuild), so you can sidekick again. Depending on your physical condition and the amount of creatine in your system, rebuilding takes anywhere from a few seconds to three minutes.

Researchers have found that supplementing with creatine monohydrate slows muscle fatigue, speeds up the rebuilding phase, and increases the total creatine content in muscles by as much as 20 to 30 percent. What this means to you is that when you consume extra creatine, you might last longer and recover faster than if you didn't take it.

Creatine as a Performance Enhancer

Here are ways to use it to increase power and add muscular bulk:

Prior to an event only   If you don't want to take creatine on a daily basis, you might consider it as a performance enhancer. Dr. Melvin Williams, a professor at the Department of Exercise Science, Physical Education and Recreation at Old Dominion University in Norfolk, Virginia says that most athletes take 20 to 25 milligrams per day for five to seven days prior to a competitive event. He believes that creatine should only be taken for the purpose of enhancing your performance in periodic competitive events, not for everyday workouts. He also says you should do a trial run with it a month or two before the competition to see how your body handles it. [30]

Daily use   There is research that disagrees with Williams, findings that show consistent use is okay, which is how most bodybuilders use it. Some researchers say daily use is preferable.

With periodic breaks   There is other research that suggests you use it for, say, two months, and then stop for a month. You won't lose any of your gains following this plan; in fact, some people say you get a bump in your progress when you resume using it.

What is best for you depends on your specific body; so you have to experiment. Consider the following:

- If you lift weights regularly, make creatine a regular supplement. Know that if you want to go off it for a month every two or three months, every authority we know says you can do so without worry of losing anything you have gained. Co-author Christensen goes off it at least twice a year and has never noticed a drop in strength or muscle mass.

- If you don't lift weights but your martial arts training involves lots of free-hand strength-developing exercises, such as pushups, pull-ups and horse stance squats, or lots of muscle straining ground grappling, you would probably benefit from ingesting creatine every day. As with bodybuilders, you can go off it for a month every two or three months without fear of losing your gains.

If your training is mostly kata and sparring, you still exercise your muscles, but not necessarily in a way that increases their bulk. Can you get by without using creatine? Yes. Might you benefit from it? We think so, and here is why.

Endurance and creatine   Some authorities say that creatine doesn't benefit endurance athletes, but we have found just the opposite. While we haven't conducted scientific research, our experiences, as well as feedback from our students and word of mouth from other martial artists, shows that creatine definitely provides more energy and endurance for those especially hard martial art workouts. Here is a study that backs up our findings.

The study, conducted by the University of Western Australia, showed that creatine could improve performance in the latter stages of such sports as field hockey, soccer and football. These aren't martial arts (though they involve lots of fighting), but their level of activity is quite similar. While numerous studies have shown that creatine helps during short periods of exercise (less than 10 minutes), the University's study set out to determine if improvements from creatine persisted into the middle and latter stages of exercise.

The researchers gathered a group of active men, though not well-trained athletes, and had them perform a series of all-out bike sprints for 80 minutes. Recovery periods of various durations were sprinkled throughout the session to mimic what occurs in soccer and field hockey. When the test was over, the men were split into two groups: One took 20 grams of creatine every day, while the other took, unbeknownst to them, a placebo (a substance that does nothing). Five days later, the men took the test again.

The group that got stuck taking a placebo didn't improve at all, but the creatine group increased their work performance by six percent, an improvement considered amazing in only five days, and outperformed their placebo group in the middle and latter

stages of the exercise test. The authors of the study concluded this: " ... the use of creatine supplementation for enhancing physical performance in multiple sprint sports (performed over a similar time frame) seems justified."

Can Creatine Hurt Your Performance?

There is some evidence that creatine might be a hindrance. For example, when cross-country runners used it, they reported that their times got worse, which might indicate that their accompanying weight gain slowed them down.

Creatine has always involved a loading phase where the user takes in about 20 grams daily for five days (though there are studies that show this is unnecessary). It's quite possible that loading creatine leads to weight gain, even several pounds. If weight gain is a concern to you, but you still want to use creatine, start out with only five grams, not 20 grams used for loading. Taking only five grams still saturates your muscles, but it takes about 30 days to do so. This extended time is okay because it provides you additional time to adjust to any weight gain. [31]

There are no known negative side affects to taking creatine supplementation. However, it may be found in 20 years that those who have been taking it for two decades may suddenly grow a third eyebrow. It does increase your trips to the restroom because for most people it acts as a diuretic the first hour after consumption. No problem as long as you replace the lost water.

Beside vitamins and minerals, we think creatine is one supplement you should use. We asked world champion kickboxing and boxer Daniella Somers if she supplemented with it, "I use protein to a lesser extent but lots of creatine as a recuperation supplement," she said. "I would certainly recommend it to others since top-level competitive sports are very demanding on your body and today's needs does not meet our needs." [32]

Note: At this writing, creatine is not considered an illegal drug. It can still be bought over the counter and the International Olympic Committee has not banned it for use by athletes.

Reduce Your Aerobic Activity to Gain Weight

Let's look at two extremes in the world of competitive running, the marathon runner and the sprinter. At their competition best, both athletes are in excellent physical shape, burn lots of calories, and yet are physically different. Why? The answer is in how they train. The marathoner has no need for large muscles, since he doesn't perform off-the-block, explosive, short duration sprints. Instead, he runs for long distances, sometimes for hours at a time. This steady, relatively slow style of running develops his slow-twitch muscle fibers, which inadvertently develops long muscles and a slender physique. However, the sprinter is usually more bulky since his running style requires explosive and powerful leg pumping movements.

Man eater One of the biggest problems of the marathoner is that he cannibalizes his own body for energy. He trains for such long periods that his body doesn't have time to refuel as well as it should to recover all the lost nutrients. So after it has exhausted all the available carbs and fats, it begins using muscle protein by means of a biochemical process that breaks the molecules of his muscles down into their basic components, amino acids, which are then used as fuel. One study found that the bodies of some runners were still cannibalizing their calves seven days after a marathon.

The point of giving you that unpleasant image is to show that long endurance training is not compatible with muscle building and weight gain. You can't simultaneously be a long distance runner and sprinter (you can, but you won't be good at either one). If you want to increase muscle mass and put on some pounds, then that should be the primary focus of your training. Don't do cardio kickboxing, stationary bicycle riding and 60-minute jogging sessions. While the martial arts does require aerobic fitness, as does a real street fight, both endeavors involve short explosions of energy, not the type developed from long periods of endurance work.

As mentioned in an earlier sidebar, if you absolutely insist on doing aerobics, limit your session to 30 minutes, three times a week.

At first the effort to gain weight slowly and carefully might seem like a major hassle, and the eroding of your patience and your growing frustration might lead you to the local bakery. But resist. Yes, some thought has to go into your diet and training program (use the log at the back of this book), but when you get the hang of it, it becomes routine and part of the whole picture that is your study of the martial arts. Once in the groove, you will wonder what it was that you thought so difficult.

Fast Facts

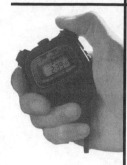

- Synergism, for our purpose here, is defined as the interaction of all training factors so that their combined effect is greater than the sum of their individual effects.

- Eating smart before training, competing or engaging in all-day seminars is an absolute must, and eating smart after training accelerates tissue repair and reenergizes the body so that it can train next time.

- The common consensus among coaches and nutritionists is that the absolute minimum time needed for basic digestion is one hour, though it's better to wait one and a half to two hours before training.

- When planning to train aerobically, your pre-training meal should consist of around 70 percent carbs, 15 percent fat and 15 percent protein.

- This training requires a big slice of pie coming from protein, roughly 35 percent, with 50 percent coming from carbs and 15 percent from fat.

- Though most seminars are non-stop training, there is the occasional pause. That's the time to take a bite of fruit, an energy bar or a chug from an energy drink.

- When you travel to the event, take some "safe" foods that you know are tolerable and provide lots of energy.

- Sugar, milk, eggs and high-protein foods should be avoided the day of the tournament since they are relatively hard to digest.

- Think of timing your eating as you do your attack when sparring: To be successful, you must choose the right technique and apply it at the right moment.

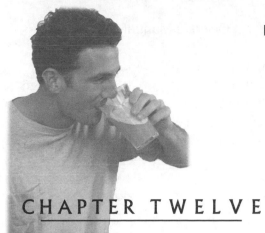

CHAPTER TWELVE

Fueling the Machine

What to Eat Before a Class, Competition or Seminar (& What Not to)

By now, it should be clear that what you eat has a significant influence on your muscle mass, weight loss effort, weight gain effort, and overall health. We have discussed how nutrition affects your training and your performance in general, but now let's get more specific and look at which foods help you get an optimum workout, to perform at your best in competition, and help you stay energized physically and mentally at one of those all-day seminars. What you eat, how much and when you eat it can make the difference between a great martial arts experience, a mediocre one or one that is just plain lousy.

A Synergistic Approach

You can work on your flexibility until your face turns blue, but if you don't pound on the heavy bags you won't learn how to get power out of those flexible techniques. While the heavy bag helps develop strong punches and kicks, if you never apply them against a live opponent in sparring, your timing, speed and distancing will never develop fully. This is because each training tool is made better when combined with others; together, they help you improve and ultimately perform at your best. The food you eat is part of this combined effort. Healthy nutrition, while good for your body, isn't enough by itself to hoist you upon the victory stand or make you the best martial artist you can be. But it becomes a powerful brick in your foundation when combined with stretching, bag work, drills, sparring and other training tools.

218 The Fighter's Body: An Owner's Manual

It's all about synergism, which for our purpose here is defined as the interaction of all these training factors so that their combined effect is greater than the sum of their individual effects.

Those Darn Kids

As a teenager, co-author Demeere thought it was natural to have to always struggle through the second hour of his class on raw nerve and willpower, and then go home completely exhausted. Having studied nutrition for several years now, it pains him to think of the training time he wasted by improperly fueling his body prior to those tough workouts, and he is amazed that he wasn't injured more than he was. He understands now that his drained energy reserves were a direct result of eating the wrong ratio of protein, carbs and fats, and too soon before his class.

Oh, but the flame of youth burns brightly Kids believe they are capable of doing anything and that they will live forever. Teenagers are especially notorious for eating poorly while at the same time inflicting tremendous stress and strain on their bodies as they dash through their busy lives. Many teens training in the martial arts are even harder on themselves. Blessed with marvelous recuperative powers, a grueling workout today is forgotten tomorrow. They believe they can do anything to their bodies and, for a while, it seems true. But the cursed clock moves forward and one day, seemingly overnight, that flame burns

less brightly. Their muscles, joints and tendons no longer tolerate the neglect and abuse that was once so mindlessly heaped upon them. They can no longer recuperate as quickly, fatigue comes sooner and body parts previously never considered, begin to hurt, and break down.

Students who ignore or can't see the obvious signs suffer the most and often drop by the wayside when the pain and effort become too great. Sadly, they are forced to stop doing what they enjoy only because they lack information. Even more sadly, many of them have the potential to continue learning, progressing and maturing into great martial artists.

Informed students, however, learn early that sleep and rest are mandatory, as is training smart and fueling the body with high-octane nutrients. The informed learn three things in particular about eating:

- Eating smart before training, competing or engaging in all-day seminars is an absolute must.

- Eating smart after training accelerates tissue repair and reenergizes the body so that it can train next time.

- Healthy eating habits are a means of keeping an edge and continuing to progress as the years and the decades pass.

Discipline

You must consciously bring that same discipline that gets you through 100 kicks in class to your decision as to what to eat in your pre-training meal. Just as you know that 100th rep makes you strong, you need to understand and accept that you must choose foods that work for you, not against you. You must convince yourself, especially those insatiable "pleasure zones" in your brain and on your tongue, that that piece of cake gives pleasure only for a couple of minutes, while a protein drink, apple and banana provide an hour of pleasure in the form of good energy to get you through a tough training session.

You understand that it's all about discipline.

*   Discipline in the kitchen means preparing your own meals, shopping for quality food, keeping track of your calories each day, learning about nutrition, and keeping a log that reveals what works for you and what doesn't.

*   Discipline means you always eat at least two hours before training or competing so the quality fuel has time to surge through your body, and it means you always refuel your engine with good nutrients after your training to speed up your recuperation.

*   Discipline means you understand that while a hamburger tastes good, you can only enjoy it on an off day,

not on a class day and never before competition.

*   Discipline means that when it comes to training, competing and all-day seminars, you eat what is necessary to be at your best, not simply to tickle your pleasure zone.

What to Eat Before

We have said repeatedly that your body's preferred source of energy comes from quality carbs, and it's especially true when considering what to eat at that all-important meal before your training, competition or seminar. You also need a little protein and fat, and we talk about that in a moment, but for now know that your best source of energy before a hard martial arts session comes from carbs. If you don't consume enough, you are going to drag.

Never fall for those diets that limit your carb intake. They don't offer anything that active people need, particularly a martial athlete needing all the energy he can get. Focus on complex, low Glycemic Index carbs that yield long-term energy, such as whole-wheat pasta, breads, beans, rice, and apples. Refer to the Glycemic Index in Chapter 3 for a complete list of the preferred low GI carbs and a list of those ugly high GI carbs that you must avoid.

"But the high GI carbs taste good," we hear students say so often. Yes, they do taste good, but what is the smart choice, the warrior choice? Is it a sugary candy bar that gives your taste buds a minute or two of pleasure, but only provides for a few minutes of energy before the bottom drops out? Or should it be quality carbs that provide long-lasting energy to support a hard training session?

When to Eat

Let's say you just consumed a whole-wheat slice of bread covered with 100 percent pure peanut butter, a pear, banana and a glass of skim milk. The moment it lands in your stomach, it's bombarded with several biochemical processes. These processes extract the nutritionally valuable particles from your food and send them throughout your body to supply you with energy, regulate your hormonal system, repair more tissue from yesterday's workout, and do a host of other things to keep you healthy and slamming those hard and fast techniques. Unusable elements in the food are extracted and sent to the trashcan, if you get our drift.

While this process takes only a minute to read, in actuality it takes much longer, up to several hours. For a routine, nontraining day, you don't need to think about it, but on your training days, when you eat in relation to your workout needs to be factored into your schedule since the digestive process is so complex. Should you eat too soon, you suffer a lack of energy and get a miserable stomach. Here is why:

Digestion requires calories Up to 10 percent of all the calories you consume are needed to digest that pear, banana, milk, and peanut butter sandwich. Problems arise when you begin training while that 10 percent is still busy fueling your digestion. In particular, complex carbohydrates, the ones needed for your kicks and punches have yet to be digested since they take the longest. Eat them too close to your practice session, and the energy won't be available when you need it the most, like when the toughest black belt in class thumps on you as if your body were one of those armless training mannequins.

Upset stomach A lack of energy may be the least of your problems should you commence training before your digestive system is through grinding up your last meal. When you pop out those backfists and sidekicks, your body shifts into high gear sending urgent blood to your muscles, accelerating your heartbeat, pumping adrenaline to where it's needed, and several other functions.

While you want all these things happening when you train or compete, it wreaks havoc on your stomach while it's still digesting your meal. Should you cut your digestion process short or force it to work with diminished resources, it will let you know it's unhappy by making you bloated and nauseous. It might even make you throw up. A lot of training partners get offended when you projectile vomit all over their training uniforms.

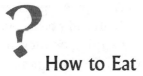

How to Eat

Let us be your mother for a moment and tell you how to eat that good food. You have a busy life, but it's important that you make every effort to eat while sitting down, rather than gobbling a burrito as you dash to your next appointment. Always keep in mind that you eat not only to rid your hunger, but to fuel your body for your day and for your training. Since the early stages of digestion begin in your mouth, it's critical to relax, kick back and chew slowly. Now, sit up and stop fidgeting!

One to two hours before The common consensus among coaches and nutritionists is that the absolute minimum time needed for basic digestion is one hour, though one and a half to two is better. Calculate your time from when you finish eating, not from when you begin. If you are a slow eater and take up to 30 minutes to finish a meal, you need to factor that in. For example if your training begins at 6 PM and you determine you need two hours for digestion, you need to begin eating at 3:30.

There are many factors involved that determine how long your body needs to digest a meal, such as your overall health, basic metabolism rate, the food consumed, and previous meals eaten that day. We suggest you start with a minimum of one hour and then add time depending on how you feel. For example, Demeere knows that he needs at least two hours to digest pasta, especially if it includes tomatoes, but he needs only an hour to digest a low-fat cheese sandwich. Christensen, through trial and error, has found that he needs two hours no matter what he eats. Experiment to see what works for you time-wise and food-wise.

Before we discuss the best foods for optimum training, let's examine the issue of food allergies and competition.

Know What Foods Don't Like You

Allergies

Your body is a miraculous machine, but it's not a perfectly engineered one. It doesn't perform at 100 percent in every area, hence the expression, "You're only human." For example, everyone has one or more types of food to which they are allergic or to which they have a low tolerance. Many children and adults are allergic to milk, though children often grow out of it. Some people are allergic to nuts, with symptoms ranging from itching, swelling and even death. Christensen knew a five-year-old girl who ate a chocolate nut cluster and died 30 minutes later. The severity of the reaction depends on the specific food, how much of it, its freshness, what other foods were eaten with it, and other factors.

Treatment is usually geared toward avoiding the "bad" foods, and taking medicine as a counter measure. Overall, allergies are treatable and don't pose an insurmountable obstacle towards a healthy lifestyle or your martial arts practice.

Note: Allergies can develop suddenly at any age. You might not know you have one now because it has yet to fully develop.

Food intolerance

Food intolerance is usually less severe than an allergic reaction. For example, people intolerant of chili and green peppers often suffer from bloating; MSG causes some to suffer from headaches and nausea; cucumbers make some people burp like a swamp frog. If you have symptoms but the cause is unclear, write down everything you eat for a week, including condiments, and then show your list to your doctor. You want the problem under control so it doesn't interfere with your training. In his book *The Science of Martial Arts Training*, Charles I. Staley suggests the following to test your personal sensitivity to certain foods.

Eat normally for a week. Note your pulse each morning when you first awaken, then right before you eat and again 15 minutes after. A significant increase (more than eight beats per minute) in the morning or after meals signals an adverse food reaction. Feeling an energy drain after eating a certain food is also an indicator.

For five days, eat only lean poultry and/or beef, fish and vegetables. Don't consume dairy products, grains or your favorite foods. Note your pulse rate when you awaken, before and after you eat, as well as any changes in your mental or physical energy.

On the sixth day, introduce dairy products. Add wheat products on the seventh day, add sugars on the eighth day and on the ninth day add anything you want (alcohol, fast food). When you introduce a food type back into your diet, say, dairy products, eat a different one at each meal, i.e., milk at breakfast, cheese at lunch and yogurt at dinner. Note your reaction to the re-introduced food and note your pulse. Report any radical reactions to your doctor.

When you complete this evaluation and know the cause of at least some of your problems, put together a diet that avoids the bad boy foods. [33]

Watch Out for Those Sneaky Blows

Okay, so you have a good looking plate of low GI, quality carbs and you are eating at 4 PM, two hours before your 6 PM class. You are doing everything right to prepare your fine-tuned fighting machine for the training to come. Good for you, but here is how you can still foul-up things.

First, be cognizant of how you prepare your food. A common error is to flavor things to the extent that they become "heavy" and hard to digest. Frying, baking and using lots of butter, margarine and vegetable oil adds substantially to the meal's fat and calorie content, making you feel sluggish and churning those lower intestines half way through your class. The best way to prepare your pre-training meal is to boil or steam your foods, methods that don't require oils, butter or margarine. Your digestive

system will love you for it, but your training partner will hate it because you will have energy to blast away at him the entire class.

Along with how you prepare your food is what you add once it's on your plate, specifically, rich sauces, salad dressings, mayonnaise, and ketchup. While some of these condiments might not be unhealthy, such as ketchup and certain oils, they digest slowly and their spices might upset your stomach during training. If you do choose to fry your food and add condiments, you should wait an additional hour or more before training to allow for proper digesting. That said, just remember that it's in your best interest to always strive to make your pre-training meal easy to digest and rich in quality carbs.

Eating for Aerobic and Anaerobic Training

When planning your diet, take into consideration whether your training will be mostly aerobic or anaerobic. Jogging, cycling, swimming, and shadowsparring moderately for 20 to 30 minutes are aerobic activities since you use the same large muscle groups somewhat rhythmically for a period of 15 minutes or longer while working at 60 to 80 percent of your maximum heart rate. However, when you kick the heavy bag as hard and fast as you can repetitiously, weight train and train for speed and explosiveness using sprints and plyometrics, you work anaerobically because the exercises involve mostly short bursts of exertion followed by periods of rest.

General, your martial arts workouts are a mix of both, such as when you go through your form 10 consecutive times or spar five, three-minute rounds, while launching your techniques hard and fast for 20 to 30 minutes. The basic movements are anaerobic (explosive, fast), but the overall activity goes longer than three minutes, thus making it aerobic. Martial arts schools that do it right combine both, though the ratio varies from school to school, depending on a host of variables, such as the particular fighting art, the school's slant (competition or self-defense) and the proficiency level of the class.

Feeding the Training Methods

Remember: Whatever type of training you do, your primary source of energy comes from carbs, though the formulas vary.

Aerobic   When planning to train aerobically, your pre-training meal should consist of around 70 percent carbs, 15 percent fat and 15 percent protein. As always, your carbs should be low GI and preferably complex ones. After your training, be sure to refill your body's energy stores by consuming good quality carbohydrates. Don't even think about a 42-ounce soda and a hotdog. Insist on good carbs, so you are replenished and raring to train again the next day.

Anaerobic   This training requires a big slice of pie coming from protein, roughly 35 percent, with 50 percent coming from carbs and 15 percent from fat. You need the building and repairing blocks of extra protein since this type of training damages your muscle tissue more than does aerobic activities. After training, refuel with both carbs and protein.

Combining them   When training aerobically and anaerobically, you want plenty of energy for the endurance training but you also want enough protein for muscle growth and repair. The popular formula, and one we like, is 60 percent carbs, 30 percent protein and 10 percent fat. For your post-exercise meal, take in 50 percent carbs, 40 percent protein and 10 percent fat to recharge your energy stores and build tired muscles. 29

As with all guidelines, these are estimated starting points and work well for most people. Still, it's important to carefully monitor how you feel from day to day. If you feel good and have sufficient energy to get through your day and your training, you don't need to change a thing. However, if you feel consistently tired or your strength is diminishing, make adjustments accordingly.

Eating on Competition Day and at Seminars

Let's put the final touches on your preparation and look at what you should eat on the very day of the event. While good nutrition can't make up for any time you wasted not training or training improperly, eating the wrong foods on the big day can definitely compound the problem. But if you have been training hard with a smart training regimen, the right choice of food can be the one additional, positive element that carries you to victory. Here are a few pointers as to how to make food work for you in today's tough competitive world.

- Eat a healthy breakfast to start your day with energy and enthusiasm for the event. You had a good night's sleep (or a restless one if you are the nervous type) and your body has gone without food for several hours. Never skip breakfast, especially on competition day. Eat at least two hours before the event, so all the nutrients have time to absorb before you perform. If your event starts early in the day, you need to get out of bed earlier than you would normally.

- Sugar, milk, eggs and high-protein foods should be avoided since they are relatively hard to digest. Instead, eat low-GI carbs such as pancakes (no syrup or butter), low-fiber fruits, fruit and vegetable juices and potatoes. [35]

- Eat every three hours but keep the meals light. As near as you can, try to determine what time you compete so you can eat accordingly. If you do your form at 11AM, eat your breakfast no later than 9 AM, though 8 AM is better. If you fight at 3 PM, try to eat a light meal right after your forms competition.

- Don't drink carbonated beverages. Most are filled with sugar and the carbonation might upset your stomach. Burping as you step into the ring is considered low class. Do drink lots of water or sports drinks throughout the day to stay well hydrated.

- Should you travel to another country to compete, avoid eating the local food two or three days before the event and never eat it on the big day. Some "foreign" foods take a while for your body to get used to and eating them might cause everything from diarrhea, abdominal pain, headaches and a host of other unpleasant reactions.

At most big international tournaments, there is food available called "Continental cuisine," meaning it's geared towards the tastes and tolerances of Westerners. Tread with caution, though, and don't automatically consider it a home-cooked meal. Some local cooks try to emulate Western food, but use local ingredients that just might come back to play havoc with your already nervous system. (Co-author Demeere once ordered french fries in China to see if there was a difference. There was: They were thick as his wrist, floating in oil and sprinkled with sugar.)

- As you train in the weeks before your competition, experiment to see how your body reacts to various foods. Determine which ones you tolerate well, which make you feel miserable and which give you the most energy. When you travel to the event, take some "safe" foods that you know are tolerable and provide lots of energy.

- Experiment with energy bars and high-carb nutrition shakes. Many competitors find them more digestible than solid foods, especially those fighters who suffer from pre-competition stress. Bars and shakes tend to be light and digest easily while still providing good energy for the events to come. Try them on your training days three or four weeks before your event to see if they might be an option for you.

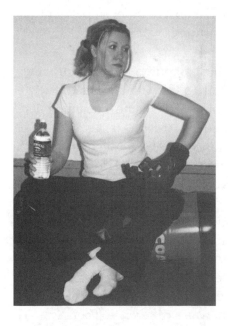

Eating at Seminars

Martial arts seminars are usually day-long sessions with one or two breaks and an hour for lunch, or less. Though these aren't ideal circumstances, you can make the best of them by following these guidelines.

- Just as when competing, it's critical to eat a nutritious and energy-producing breakfast to prepare you for the long day of training and learning.

- Eat lightly and eat for energy. Though most seminars are non-stop training, there is always the occasional pause in the action for whatever reason. That is the time to take a bite of fruit, an energy bar or a chug from an energy drink.

- During lunch, eat a meal comprised mainly of low GI carbs and foods low in fat. This keeps your blood sugar stable for a longer period, preventing your energy from fluctuating.

- Avoid soft drinks or coffee at lunch, as they can dehydrate you, something you don't need when training hard and sweating profusely. Instead, drink water or a sports drink. Keeping your body hydrated is vital to your performance and health.

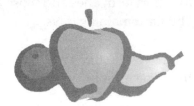

Use Your Warrior Spirit

Eating correctly before, during and after a martial arts competition or seminar takes a little extra time and sometimes a whole lot of discipline. There is no getting around this. However, as a smart, informed martial artist, you know that to fuel your muscles, tendons, tissues, skeletal system, blood, and brain properly before and after a tough martial arts session, you need the right combination of protein, carbs, and fat, all consumed at the right time. Think of timing your eating as you do your attack when sparring: To be successful, you must choose the right technique and apply it at the right moment.

Knowing this is one thing; applying it takes a warrior spirit.

Fast Facts

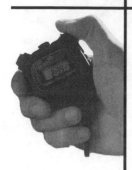

- Does not being sick automatically mean you are healthy? No. Such thinking is mediocre, and as a martial artist striving to be the best you can be, you should never settle for mediocrity, especially when it comes to your health.

- The less time you spend sick, the more time you have to train.

- While nutritious food and supplements are critical to your long-term training and wellness plan, you also need to make a dedicated effort to avoid injury, short term ones and those that come back to haunt you for all your remaining days.

- You are at risk when day after day you do the same drills and the same exercises, working the same muscles, joints and tendons.

- Macrocycle training begins with a general long-term strategy and then breaks down to a day-to-day strategy. You decide on whatever goal you want for the season and then form your training schedule into progressive stages.

- Know and accept that it's okay to lose a little of your conditioning and competitive edge when you take a week or two off. It's considerably more important to heal all the small and big injuries and allow your brain to relax.

- If you go into every class worrying about getting hurt, you are going to get hurt. It's a better mindset to accept the possibility that you might get injured in training, and then do everything you can to minimize that possibility.

- Learn how to listen to your body, which is done by making a conscious effort to develop a dialog between it and your mind, a communication sometimes referred to as "physical conscience."

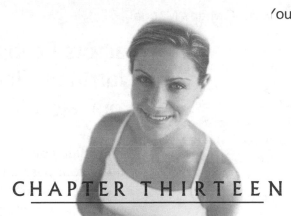

CHAPTER THIRTEEN

Your Long-Term Plan

Don't Settle for Just Feeling Okay

Most people think of good health as feeling well and rarely suffering from illness. This is correct, but barely. When you have been slammed hard by the flu bug, struggling out from under your fever-damp sheets makes the labors of Hercules pale in comparison. You sway dizzily for a long moment and then stumble and stagger to the bathroom, wanting only to return to bed and die peacefully in a drug-induced sleep. But you survive and a week later you marvel at how wonderful it feels to be well: "Aaah, the flu is gone and I'm healthy again."

Oh really? Does not being sick automatically mean you are healthy? No. Such thinking is mediocre, and as a martial artist striving to be the best you can be, you should never settle for mediocrity, especially when it comes to your health. Understand this: There is much more to good health and feeling great than not being sick. Consider the simple scale below:

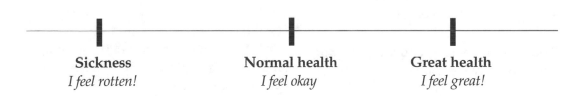

Sickness	Normal health	Great health
I feel rotten!	*I feel okay*	*I feel great!*

Most people live their lives in the middle of this scale. Some do just enough to avoid sliding to the far left where there is sickness and disease, while others don't do anything more than just hope they don't slide to the left. When asked how they feel, they shrug and say, "I feel okay, I guess." They haven't a clue that there is a better life to the far right, a world of great health, zest, energy and a powerful, positive outlook. To use a cliché: a place where they feel like a million bucks.

When you live on the right side of the scale, you bounce through your day with the energy of three people and tackle life and all that it throws at you with an extraordinary, positive outlook. It's an indescribably wonderful place that is far superior to the center of the scale where people just feel okay. For them, the slightest problem, a sick family member or a poor night's sleep, nudges them to the left, maybe all the way. But by living on the far right side, that germ-carrying family member, that bad night's sleep (that plague carrying rat) just bounces off you, or at the most moves you a little toward the center. This is because the far right side provides an extra buffer against sickness so that it takes more to move you to the far left than it does the person living in the center. Here is a simple bumper sticker for you:

The less time you spend sick, the more time you have to train.

Factors Beyond Nutrition That Affect Your Health

While quality nutrition is vital to solidify your position on the right side of the scale, it's important that you also consider factors beyond diet. Though this book is primarily about nutrition and healthy training, there is much more to having optimum health and a strong, mostly injury-free body for all your life. Actually, there are so many factors that it would take volumes to list them all, and it's an on-going list, as every day something new is discovered that is good for us as well as bad for us.

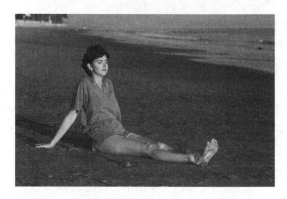

Many negative influences are out of our control — terrorism, earthquakes, typhoons — while others are quite easy to change or modify. For example, studies show that living next to a busy airport impacts your long-term good health due to sound pollution disturbing your sleep. While you can't make the airport move somewhere else, you do have control over where you live.

Examine your life to see what negative influences on your health can be changed, even if it takes effort. Here are a few aspects to living that tear people down over time:

• Negative co-workers
• Bad boss
• Bad marriage
• Long commute
• Living next to a freeway
• Poor social life
• Too many commitments
• Working two jobs
• Nagging injury
• Terrible neighbors
• Late hours
• Lost TV remote

Minimizing Injury

While nutritious food and supplements are critical to your long-term training and wellness plan, you also need to make a dedicated effort to avoid injury, short term ones and those that come back to haunt you for all your remaining days. Let's look at just a few things under your control that keep your body well as you push yourself through the rigors of strenuous martial arts training in the years to come.

The way your authors began in the martial arts is now considered "old school." We trained virtually every day in classes that pushed us past the point of exhaustion, where hard contact, including broken bones, were the norm and bumps and bruises were no big deal. We did endless repetitions of basic techniques, stances and footwork, and

forms were done a dozen times on an easy night, and always with the teacher hitting us with a stick or fist every time we erred. At the end of class, when our bodies were limp with exhaustion, we sparred with minimum or no protective gear. Sprained knees, a wrenched neck, broken fingers and toes, and chipped teeth were routine and accepted as symbols of our warriorhood. (Yes, we sound like your grandparents who claim they trudged five miles through snow to school every day, but unlike them we aren't lying to you.) We loved it, though, and we kept coming back for more, while other students dropped out. Some left after just a few weeks because of the rigors and monotony of the training, while others stayed for a year or two, eventually leaving because of the hard contact and small, and sometimes big, training injuries in nearly every class.

Overtraining

Injuries were only part of the risk. The bigger danger came from nonstop hard training. Nearly every day we put our muscles and tendons through grueling workouts, only to do the same drills and exercises the next day before our bodies had recuperated fully from the last session. Then we did it again the next day. If you had looked up "overtraining" in the dictionary back then, you would have found a picture of us punching, kicking and sweating.

Even the strongest can take only so much of this before something snaps or breaks off. You know you have been overdoing it when someone on the street runs up to you from behind, and says, "I think you dropped this." And it's your elbow.

Diversify Your Training

During our early years, many hard training students with great potential dropped out because they were worried about getting injured or were debilitated by old injuries that kept haunting them. Don't let this happen to you. Even if your training isn't as knock down and bruising as was ours, you are still at risk when day after day you do the same drills and the same exercises, working the same muscles, joints and tendons. Repetition is important, but to last in the martial arts for many years, and do so healthily, you need to find ways to train so your body stays intact and your enthusiasm stays high.

The martial arts are a great way to stay healthy throughout your life, but not if you push your body to the breaking point.

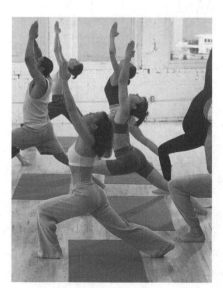

Periodization

While the old school training method did give us a tough mindset, there are other ways to achieve the same thing and do so without all the pain and injury (don't even get us started about our surgery scars), and keep the dropout rate to a minimum. A concept called periodization involves cycling the intensity of your training volume and the specific drills and exercises you do. Although it's relatively new to the martial arts, it's a training methodology that has been used in other sports for decades

Periodization was born after sport scientists discovered two critical aspects about physical training:

- Training as hard as you can and for as long as you can gives you maximum result in about four to six weeks.

- Should you continue at the same pace after four to six weeks, your progress slows and then reverses. Reverses! There comes a point in your hard training when you cross an invisible line and begin to suffer from reduced energy, strength, skill, and endurance. That is when injury rears its ugly head.

Macro, Meso and Micro Training

This is a highly effective way to periodize your training for optimum progress and minimum risk to your muscles, tendons, ligaments and bones. It begins with the general overall plan called the macrocycle.

Macrocycle Macrocycle is a self-imposed timeframe, anywhere from five months to a year, and is further divided into a preparatory phase, competitive phase and transition phase. Here is what occurs in each:

- The preparatory phase lays a foundation by developing strength, skill and endurance specific to your fighting art.

- The competitive phase is designed to maintain the attributes built in the preparatory phase while at the same time polishing the pertinent technical skills.

- The transition phase is when you get to rest, allowing your body to heal from injuries, your energy reserve to refill and your mind to relax from your rigid training discipline. Some athletes rest completely during this time, while others train lightly or play another sport for a while.

You don't need to be a competitor to use periodization. Maybe you want to prepare for a belt exam or get in shape for several high-intensity, weekend seminars during the year. Even if your only goal is to train properly and become a better martial artist, cycling your training is a highly effective and scientific way to progress.

How to Make It Work for You

As just described, macrocycling begins with a general long-term strategy and then breaks down to a day-to-day strategy. You decide on whatever goal you want for the season and then form your training schedule into progressive stages. You can go into great detail if you like, writing down minute by minute what you plan to do each day, each week and each month, or you can keep it general and go with the flow. What is important is that you find a format with which you are comfortable.

Even the most rigid schedule should allow you to adapt to any of life's surprises. Say you receive a small injury during the second week of the preparatory phase. Although you are scheduled to train intensely, the injury

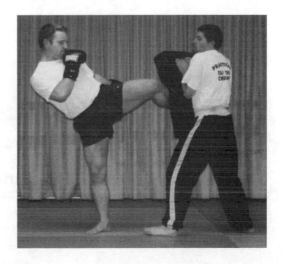

forces you to slow down to a moderate pace for several sessions. Two weeks later you are healed enough to resume hard training, which means you need to adjust your schedule to play catch up. Be careful you don't over train or get hurt again in your zest to get back on track. Know that you can't make up for the two weeks of intense training you lost, but if you push yourself a little, eat healthily and get plenty of rest, you can minimize the lost time and lack of progress. It's all made possible by your carefully organized, yet flexible training schedule. Remember, the objective is to make it work for you, not for you to become a slave to it.

Let's say you want to be in top condition for two upcoming tournaments. The first one is to be held the first weekend in April and the other a couple of weekends later. This is a perfect situation for macrocycle, mesocycle, and microcycle training schedules. Here is one way to do it:

Macrocycle

Preparatory Phase   For the first two months (January and February for our purposes here), you work on basic conditioning exercises to build a solid base for what is to come. Increase your cardiovascular system by running, swimming, cycling, shadowsparring, or bag work, and increase your strength and explosiveness by working hard with weights or increasing the intensity of your dynamic tension exercise. Push your flexibility training to add speed and range to your techniques and reduce injury potential. All your basic techniques — straight punches, backfists, front kicks, roundhouse kicks, sidekicks and footwork— are practiced repetitiously to increase speed, power and accuracy. Work on any weak areas until they are no longer weak.

The emphasis during this period is on volume of training, up to two hours each session and up to six days a week. The volume is high (amount of training, length of sessions and number of sessions each week), but the intensity (how hard you train) is low. The general rule is that when the volume goes up, the intensity goes down and vice versa. If you were to increase the volume and intensity, you would risk overtraining, which is what this training concept is designed to prevent.

Sample Macrocycle:

Preparatory Phase		Competitive Phase		Transition Phase
January	February	March	April	May

Competitive Phase Now you are into the third month, March, a time to transfer your basic conditioning and skill training from the first phase into specific, point-winning techniques for the tournaments, while maintaining all that you have gained thus far. You spar frequently, work combinations in the mirror and against a partner, and thump the heavy bag to keep your power and cardio system in top condition. Since tournament fighting is done in spurts, clashes lasting only a few seconds, anaerobic conditioning becomes key during this phase. Your training consists of three to five all-out days, with sessions no longer than 90 minutes. This phase lasts three weeks.

Tapering Phase The tapering phase begins the final week of March as you near the end of the Competitive Phase, with a week to go before the first tournament. Tapering is based on the principle of "super compensation," which is discussed later in this chapter. For now, know that for these seven days, you reduce your training to recuperate as much as possible from the intense workouts done up to this point, so you are raring to go on D-day.

Decrease the volume of training to about 30 minutes a session, but keep the intensity high as if you were in the ring fighting to break a tie. You want to maintain your peak aerobic and anaerobic fitness but allow your muscles and joints to rest a little before the tournament. While reducing the workload the week before competition might seem unusual, it's a proven strategy that ensures optimal physical

performance in any sport. In a nutshell, it allows your strength, endurance and technical skills to peak on the day you need them.

Now, if you were only competing in one Saturday tournament, Sunday would begin your transition phase, a time to let your trashed body get some much needed rest. However, since you want to compete in another tournament in three weeks, you get to rest only three days. On Wednesday, you begin two weeks of competition-oriented workouts designed to strengthen your aerobic and anaerobic conditioning, sharpen your sparring skills, and work combinations in the mirror and on a training partner, sessions lasting no more than 90 minutes. Reduce your sessions to 30 minutes a week out from the tournament, but train hard as if you were in the ring. Take Friday off from training and spend time visualizing yourself excepting the trophy. Saturday, you are ready to go.

Transition Phase Congratulations, you made it to the transition phase. The tournaments are over, your walls are lined with trophies, and now you can reward yourself for all that hard work with loads of pie, cake, and pizza. Hey, get back here! We are kidding. But you do get to give your body a break and let it recuperate from the volume and intensity of training that has taken a toll on you, even if you don't actually feel it.

We know it's not considered macho in some circles, but you should rest for a few days, even a week, and take it easy when you do resume training. Know and accept that it's okay to lose a little of your conditioning and competitive edge, as it's considerably more important to heal all the small and big injuries and allow your brain to relax. Once your body has recovered fully, you can resume normal training, or start another macrocycle.

Note: There should be a smooth transition from the first phase to the second phase, and from the rest phase back into the preparatory phase. Don't, for example, end the preparatory phase on one day and then start the competitive phase going all out the following day. The sage says, "Everything in moderation." Over a period of a week, gradually decrease the preparatory phase training as you add exercises in the competitive phase. This gradual approach has been found to yield the best results and is the least harmful to your body.

Mesocycle

Once you have determined in general what you want to work on in the preparatory and competitive phases of your macrocycle, you can break down your training into specifics to know exactly what you are going to do each month in both phases. This process is called the mesocycle. Below is one possible mesocycle for your preparatory phase, using a week-by-week schedule.

Notice that the first week of training is easy compared to Week Four. In Week One, there is only one day when you have to combine, say, martial arts with endurance training, or strength training with endurance, leaving the rest of the week for one type of training per day. In Week Two, there are two days when you do two types of training, say, jog before breakfast and martial arts training in the evening. As you progress through the weeks, more and more days require two types of training. Also, each week requires that you lift slightly heavier weights or do a little more dynamic tension, run a little faster and kick the bag a little harder (see why rest is so critical?). This progression

Sample Mesocycle:

Week 1	Week 2	Week 3	Week 4
Strength training: 2 days	Strength training: 2 days	Strength training: 3 days	Strength training: 4 days
Endurance: 2 days	Endurance: 3 days	Endurance: 3 days	Endurance: 4 days
Martial arts: 3 days	Martial arts: 3 days	Martial arts: 4 days	Martial arts: 4 days

continues through the weeks up to Week Four, where you do an incredible volume of training. It's doable, though, because you have worked up to it progressively.

The second month Your mesocycle for the second month of preparatory training is virtually the same as the first except that the overall intensity is increased. Consider your needs as to how you want to do this. One way is to follow Week Four's schedule, but gradually increase the intensity of the strength, endurance, and martial arts training each week throughout the second month. At the same time, you want to increase the volume of your martial arts training. For example, if your training has been, say, 60 percent martial arts, 20 percent weights and 20 percent cardio during the first month, up your martial arts training to 70 percent, and drop your cardio and strength training to 15 percent each. Although you change the percentages, the overall volume remains the same; the intensity, however, goes up. You might find the best way to accomplish this is by going harder and faster in your drills and sparring tougher opponents.

Microcycle

When you microcycle, you break down your training even further so you know what you are going to do for your strength workout, endurance workout and your martial arts workout. Below is a one-week example of the above mesocycle.

If you like to follow a rigid training schedule, you can break this down even further by listing the exact exercises, drills, endurance times or distance, and the types and exact number of basic punches and kicks.

Our micro sample shows one way to combine different types of training into small, manageable blocks throughout the week. Make a similar plan for every week to ensure that your training allows you to systematically increase the intensity in the preparatory phase. Now, if by the end of your second week you find that you are overly tired, check your microcycle schedule to see if maybe you have increased too quickly or written down more than you can recuperate from. Can you see how writing it down helps you to see at a glance where the problems are?

Sample Microcycle:

Monday	Tuesday	Wednesday	Thursday	Friday	Saturday	Sunday
Strength: Upper body Martial arts: Basic punches	Endurance: Jogging or Shadow-sparring	Martial arts: Basic kicks	Strength: Lower body	Endurance: Jogging or Shadow-sparring	Martial arts: Basic combina-tions	Rest

Is this a tough training regimen? Oh yes. You can do it, though, because it's progressive, you fuel your body with high-octane nutrients and because you get plenty of shuteye. Here are a couple of points about periodization for you to ponder as you begin to work with it:

- Few athletes construct a perfect periodization plan their first time out. If yours has some rough spots, don't worry about it. With a little trial and error you will find a plan that is tailor made for your needs, though even then it requires continuous refinement. Consider the information provided here a good, solid base from which to begin. Since the subject is extensive and beyond the scope of this book, we encourage you to research further. Begin with the writings of Dr. Tudor O. Bompa. Not only does he have a wonderful name, he is considered the foremost expert on periodization. The bottom line is this: Periodization works for top athletes, and it will work for you, too, whether you use it for competition or as a proven way to get into top shape.

- The Russians have a unique doll that is designed somewhat like this program. You open the main doll, and there is another. Open that one and there is one more. The further you go, the more dolls you find. Think of macro as the main doll, and within it are smaller ones: the meso and micro; all interconnected.

Note   To reiterate, make sure throughout these cycles that you eat as healthily as you can. It's vastly important that you fuel your body with high quality nutrition to help you through these grueling workouts and then recuperate afterwards to face tomorrow's training.

Versatile and Safe

The macrocycle, mesocycle and microcycle approach to training is an excellent way to lose weight, prepare for a belt exam, demonstration or to simply cycle your training throughout the year. Proper use of these cycles helps to keep your training interesting, prevent over training and keep your body healthy over the long haul.

More on Preventing Injury

Several years ago, a study of sport injuries per season showed soccer to be the top scorer while boxing, judo and karate fell near the bottom of the long list. A second list ranking the severity of injuries per sport placed martial arts near the top, while soccer scored near the bottom. This leads to the conclusion that you are more likely to get injured playing soccer (not counting the bloody riots in the bleachers) than you are getting injured in a karate or judo class. However, when you do get hurt in the martial arts, it's more apt to require professional medical treatment and surgery than those injuries received when kicking a ball around on a field.

This shouldn't surprise anyone. The martial arts are all about self-control as you train with others in sometimes emotionally volatile sessions. Teachers enforce rules to ensure everyone trains and learns in an environment that is as safe as possible, with an emphasis on mutual respect, symbolized by the exchange of salutes or bows: *May I learn from you and you from me, and may our training be safe.* Nonetheless, you aren't studying flower arranging, but rather an activity where you purposefully launch powerful kicks and punches at your opponent. You train to overwhelm him, hurt him, escape from him, and when it's sport, to score a point on him with a hard, fast and controlled blow. What is considered foul play in other sports is the singular goal in the martial arts. So even with all the precautions, injuries still happen, and when they do, the potential for serious injury is inherently greater than in most other physical activities.

To work around this, you need to first accept the risks but not dwell on them. If you think about every step as you jog up a set of stairs, you fall. Likewise, if you go into every class worrying about getting hurt, you are going to get hurt. It's a better mindset to accept the possibility that you might get injured in training, and then do everything you can to minimize that possibility.

If avoidance of the risk isn't possible — for example, your class is working on over-the-shoulder judo throws — your skill, knowledge and preparation go a long ways toward getting you through the drill in one piece, though that one piece might be a little jarred. Now, if you perceive pain as just pain, similar future exercises might be feared. To avoid being afraid and to grow as a martial artist and a warrior, you must view pain as important feedback data that you did something wrong or that the technique, though you did everything right, is one that hurts no matter what precautions you take.

How Your Authors Learned the Hard Way

When co-author Demeere began training for competitive fighting he discovered that one of his best weapons was the muay Thai roundhouse kick. He liked it because of its speed, power and versatility, and he liked kicking with his shin rather than his foot. He worked it hard on the heavy bag, and though he toughened his legs to some degree, it was not enough to tolerate the acute pain of connecting with an opponent's pointy elbows and bony knees. The blocks were often so debilitating that he would hobble home after class to apply ice packs to his swollen shins and ankles. After a few of these painful training sessions, he avoided using the kick, which frustrated him because he had trained hard to make it one of his best.

After pondering the situation for a few days, Demeere began to see the kick and its vulnerability differently. He discovered that his fear of pain had kept him from kicking with full power and speed, which gave his sparring partner time to block. By applying more mental energy into setting up the attack correctly — looking for the right openings, using precision timing and developing laser-like accuracy — Demeere stopped thinking about the possibility of pain and concentrated more intensely on execution. While he still received the fun-filled elbow and knee into his shinbone, it happened only once every few weeks, as opposed to every night.

Co-author Christensen says he has been cursed with long fingers and long toes, good for swinging through the jungle, but bad when left unprotected in the martial arts. When he began training in the mid-1960s, there was little in the way of protective equipment. Sprained and broken fingers and toes were almost a constant companion in those days, so students either stayed home with their injuries or came to class and tried to find ways to train around them. Christensen's method was to refrain from using the injured part no matter what the drill. If he had a right thumb in a splint, he held it behind his back as he worked only with his left hand on drills, bag work and sparring. If he trashed a toe, he wouldn't kick with the injured foot, and if it hurt to put his weight on it when kicking with the good one, he stopped kicking all together and worked his punches.

The happy result of working around his injuries was that he never missed a workout, he grew stronger in his hand techniques when his kicks were out of commission, stronger in his kicks when his hands were hurt, and he learned what he could and couldn't do when he had a debilitating injury. This paid off for him several times in his duties as a police officer when he got injured fighting a resisting suspect but had to stay in the battle until he had the person under control.

Injuries Hamper Your Progress

Injury prevention should be an ongoing quest in your training. With each injury, you lose valuable, synergistic training when you have to work around it, and in the long run, cumulative injuries can lead to permanent problems. Christensen has a knee, finger, lower back and toe that have never completely healed over the years. The back injury happened over 35 years ago, the toe 20 years ago and today he still has to work around them.

It doesn't have to be this way because today we have more and better information as to how to train intelligently.

Common sense ways to avoid injury
The more you know about a subject, the more options you have to work with it, confront it and even make it go away. Here are a few simple precautions that won't hinder your martial arts training

but will help you to train smarter and safer to stay in it for the long run.

- Warm up and cool down. Never gloss over a good warm-up in your eagerness to begin training. Your body needs to transition gradually into strenuous training; to omit it is in an invitation to injury. Cooling down after your training helps your muscles recuperate and helps to prevent stiffness.

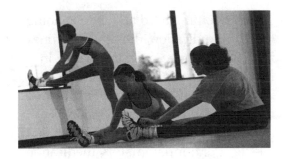

- Be cautious with certain so-called toughening and hardening exercises, such as beating yourself with sticks, kicking iron poles with your shins and beating your knuckles on cement (and stabbing your eyes with a fork). If you aren't sure about such training, tell your teacher that you want to consult your doctor before you participate. It's just smart to make an informed decision before risking irreparable damage to your one and only body. If you insist on such exercises of questionable value, please proceed gradually.

- Flexibility is important at any age for all martial artists, and it's especially important for the older fighter. It's vital that you stay supple and limber for the specifics of martial arts training and to reduce the risk of being forced beyond your range. Avoid dangerous stretching methods, such as ballistic stretching (bouncing while you stretch) or dropping into the splits without a warm-up. Yes, some people can do these things without getting hurt, but it's not worth the risk. If you persist, pray that that *riiiip* sound is your pants, not those oh-so-precious groin muscles.

- Be careful of excessive contact. Some schools slam home punches and kicks with such force that the training is just short of a real fight, a practice that is highly dangerous and conducive to injury. For best results, train with light contact to the head and medium to the body, while both parties wear protective equipment. Try to match yourself with others whose thoughts on contact match yours. Only when you and your instructor or coach are convinced that your training has reached a point where you can handle full contact should you venture into that arena.

Listen to Your Body

When you have been training consistently for a year or two, you develop an ability to almost hear your body speak to you.

"Dude, headbutts on that old, hard canvas bag hurts my forehead. Find a Nerf bag, pleeeease. "

"Hey man, I don't like it when you don't warm-up. Can you feel my hamstring getting ready to pop?"

"Yo, Bozo. How do you like that piercing pain in your wrist? Maybe next time you should make a better fist before hitting the hand-held pads."

The trick is to learn how to listen, which is done by making a conscious effort to develop a dialog between your body and your mind, a communication sometimes referred to as "physical conscience." This means you are in tune with the meaning of certain feelings, sensations and reactions that your body sends to your brain. There is nothing mystical about this (unless the voice you hear is coming from a tiny fairy sitting on a leaf); you are already familiar with such simple inner dialog that says you are hungry, tired and sick. With just a little effort, you begin to understand what your body is telling you regarding food, fluids, rest, muscle strain, and sore joints.

When Demeere combines a week of extreme training with a week of poor sleep he gets a warning in his knees and in a shoulder, a strange tingling sensation that tells him he is doing too much. If he ignores these feelings, a long-time rotator cuff injury comes calling and his trick knees make him walk all funny like. Even with plenty of sleep, he knows that should he train too hard, he is visited by an old hamstring injury. He knows all this because he is in tune with his body, and as such, he knows just how far to go before pain and injury come visiting with their red-hot pokers.

There is nothing hard about developing this communication, though sometimes it takes a nudge to open the dialog. In Demeere's case, it took the third reoccurrence of a rotator cuff problem in one year to get the conversation rolling. Since getting a big, chrome needle of anti-inflammatory medication injected deeply into the shoulder joint ranks in the top 10 experiences that aren't fun, he now listens to his body. He tries to get sufficient sleep, plans his workouts better and listens carefully to warnings from his body.

With a little effort, you too can hear your body's warning and know which sensations are small nuisances and which are potentially serious medical problems. When you have reached that point of self-knowledge — it doesn't take long and it isn't difficult— you will enjoy more injury-free training days.

When You Need More Than an Apple a Day

Say you have been listening to your body and it's been telling you that it needs something more than just rest or a few easy workouts. It needs — a doctor! Nooo! We know very well how martial artists hate to visit doctors. Christensen has to be dragged kicking and screaming to an appointment, as he whines, "That mean, perverted man always pokes and pries and peers into places on me where the sun never reaches."

While Christensen hates doctors because he is a coward, other fighters refuse to see one because they perceive it as somehow not befitting of their tough image. They believe that warriors should just eat the pain and keep on fighting. Well, this isn't wise. In fact, it's dumb. While you don't need to visit the doc every time you get a bruise, you do need to go when your body tells you to. When the message it sends makes you feel uneasy, don't ignore it. Listen to it. Take an hour out of one day and have the doc check it just to be sure.

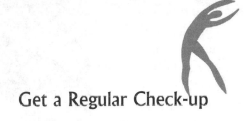

Get a Regular Check-up

Getting an extensive medical check up once a year should be part of your long-term health plan. Once you hit the big 4-0, consider checking with a doctor every six months. With today's medical technology, a simple blood test can reveal a host of illnesses at an early stage. What was untraceable five years ago can now be detected instantly on a standard test. As we were working on this book, a friend of Christensen's was given just a few weeks to live because he waited too long for a checkup (he died just before we finished). Visiting the doctor is not something you should fear and postpone, but embrace into your lifestyle.

Regular checkups increase the likelihood that your life will be long and healthy.

Rest

Many of the same fighters who refuse to go to a doctor look at rest as only for sissies. "I'll get all the sleep I need when I'm dead," some say. Or, " Five hours of sleep is all I ever need." Well, it's tough to contest the "when I'm dead" argument, but science doesn't agree that five hours is enough sleep. New studies continually show that you need seven to eight hours after stressing your body with vigorous physical activity, such as martial arts training. The reason, and we have said it before, is this: It's not the training that makes you stronger and faster, but the rest and sleep you get afterwards.

Hard training drains your reserves, damages muscle tissue, and depletes your energy. When it's over, your body begins to refill those energy reserves and repair your muscles (which happens quickly when you eat properly afterwards). If you train and rest smart, your refreshed body develops a little more strength, endurance and speed than you had before your last training session. This amazing process is called "super-compensation."

Super-compensation   In simple terms, this means that your body doesn't like to be worn down in training, so it adapts by growing just a little stronger and faster, and building a slightly larger supply of energy. Once you have done, say, two or three more workouts that are exactly the same, your body doesn't need to adapt, so it no longer super-compensates. By always training the same way, you hit a plateau, meaning you no longer progress. To continue to super-compensate, you need to give your body new stimulus by way of intensity, content and volume of training.

Should you stop training for a month or longer and there is no stimulus to your body, the higher levels of strength and endurance you achieved drop back to their original levels (and if you didn't reduce your calories during this time-off period, you begin to get pudgy). Fortunately, the diminished training and resultant loss of energy, strength and endurance don't happen overnight and it's not irreversible. As we have noted before, it's good for you to rest or reduce the volume and intensity of your training occasionally so you can recuperate physically and refresh mentally. Just don't go too long. The old bodybuilding cliché "use it or lose it" applies here, too.

Train again at the peak of your recuperation   The ideal time to train after your last workout is the moment your recuperation is complete and just before the extra energy the super-compensation created begins to dissipate. It's a place some athletes call the "sweet spot." Should you train again before your body has fully recuperated from the last workout, you risk injury from overtraining, but if you wait too long, that extra energy diminishes to where it was before you began. The good news is that it's a fairly large window of opportunity, so it's not the end of the world should you miss one workout. Miss three or four, though, or let your training schedule get erratic, and you take the "super" out of super-compensation since you aren't building on the last compensation. For instance, when you train on Monday your body super compensates and is usually ready for another workout on Wednesday. Should you skip Wednesday's and not train again until Saturday, the benefits from Monday's workout have already dissipated and you are back to where you were before Monday's training. [36] [37]

How long it takes before your body finds that place where you are fully recovered and your energy reserve hasn't begun to drop back to its original level depends on your overall fitness, the type of training you did, the intensity, your age, and other factors. Experience and your ability to listen to your body go a long way toward helping you zero in on the right moment.

The secret: sleep   The easiest way to increase the odds of finding that sweet spot is to sleep well. Try for a solid eight hours, an amount that ensures that your body gets enough rest to recuperate fully from the rigors of training. Oh yes, eating correctly is half of the equation:

Ample rest + high-octane fuel = the sweet spot.

When life interferes   We all know that life has a way of interfering with our plans, and sometimes we have no choice but to train without sufficient rest. It can be done, but you must tread softly. Here are two examples, one that shows how to do it right and one that shows the wrong way. First the right approach:

While writing this book, Demeere's second child entered the world kicking and punching (Demeere swears the boy did a pretty good kata an hour after being born), which brings forth another equation: newborn = no sleep for parents. Month after month, the Demeeres suffered from low-quality sleep or none at all. Though the father couldn't train as hard as was his norm, he did manage to train sufficiently to stay in condition while not stressing his body to a place where it was at risk of breaking. He managed this because he was in tune with himself: He understood the risk, knew the importance of eating properly and understood that he had to train within the limits of his fatigue, sleep deprivation and reduced recuperation.

Demeere did it the right way; here is an example of the wrong way:

Several years ago, co-author Christensen worked the 4 PM to midnight shift on the police department and then taught three karate classes every morning. At one point, he had grown deeply fatigued from weeks of late calls to 2 AM and the accompanying adrenaline rush that prevented him from falling asleep before dawn. Still, he had to get up at 8 AM and be at his school ready to instruct the 9 AM class. Although only 25 years old and in top condition, something had to give from this grueling schedule. One day as he launched a spinning hook kick, the kneecap in his stationary leg ripped loose, tearing a path through muscle and tendon. Though he had major surgery followed by months of physical therapy, today, years later, cold winter days nestle cruelly in his knee, reminding him of his error.

Understand how you respond to different training   Along with learning to listen to your body is the ability to differentiate between a class that gives you a bit of soreness in the morning and one that has you moaning in agony when the sun first peaks through your bedroom curtains. Knowing how your body reacts to, say, a kata class versus a sparring class gives you direction as to how much sleep you need that night. If you know you have to get up extra early tomorrow morning, take it easy in class tonight, but if you know you can sleep past breakfast tomorrow, push yourself a little. Once you get in tune with your body and understand its relationship to various types of training, many more good days will be yours, and your progress will happily astound you.

A Final Word on Machismo

In our early years in the martial arts, we trained long and hard, and not just a little insanely. Did we get mentally and physically tough by training beyond our limits? Yes, but it came at a cost, as we now have scars and lingering injuries to remind us of those times.

Today, we still train hard but not stupidly. We exercise with a learned wisdom, one that understands the limitations of the human body and one that knows safer paths to mental and physical toughness. Now when we get an injury, we don't "work through it" (whatever the heck that means), but we train around it, stop and treat it or let it rest for a few days. Once it's healed, and only after it's completely healed, do we resume our normal training.

Is this considered macho in some circles? Probably not. Do we care? Not even a little. We have been in that macho circle and we have seen what it does to fighters' bodies. We have permanent injuries of our own, but we are lucky in that we can still train, though painful reminders will always be with us.

Today, our goal is probably the same as yours, which is to live and train long and healthily with few permanent injuries. We have come to the conclusion that the macho way isn't worth spending the last third of our lives (or longer) with pain and debilitation. Hopefully, you see it that way, too.

Fast Facts

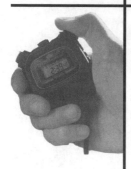

- *What doesn't kill you makes you stronger* - Nietzsche

- Before eating that taste treat, that momentary taste treat, think: "Yes, it will taste good...but only for a few seconds. To burn it off, I'll have to jog for an hour, or kick the bag for 45 minutes.

- An occasional relapse is inevitable, but don't use it as an excuse to go off your plan.

- When sick, eat quality nutrients to make war with the virus and stretch a little to get your blood flowing and loosen your muscles.

- Just as alcoholics have to learn that they can have a good time with friends and family without getting drunk, we too need to accept the fact that we can have a nice time without stuffing ourselves with junk that is harmful to our health and training.

- Why not make it a goal to be as healthy as possible this date next year, and a long-term goal to be as healthy as possible this date 10 years from now? If you are going to be around anyway, why not be as healthy as you can?

- Self-talk has been used successfully in athletics for many years. Super achievers in the sports world as well as those in endeavors outside of it have found it to be a powerful tool that helps them achieve their goals

- Just as proper nutrition is half the battle in your training strategy, mental commitment — getting your head on right — is half the battle in staying on course.

- You must be alert for rough spots and then do what you have to do when they appear so you can keep going.

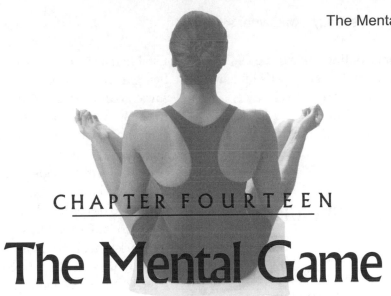

CHAPTER FOURTEEN

The Mental Game

Probably more fighters find a training schedule easier to maintain than following a healthy eating regimen, especially since eating often encompasses one's emotional state. For example, many people eat cake to make them feel happier, drink a beer to feel less tense and munch a bag of Fritos to help fight the boredom of watching television on Saturday night. While there is some psychological comfort in these foods, the effect is only temporary and soon the brain seeks more comfort food, and more, and...

To combat these urges, you need an ironclad discipline in place to act as a guard against temptation. At first, you might hesitate to block that ice cream treat, but with a longing sigh, you do the right thing and swat it aside. You might even drop your guard when you see that second piece of pizza, but at the last moment, you snap out a block. Yes, it's hard to be so defensive, but trust us when we say that it does get easier with

each passing day. Here are a couple of bumper stickers for you.

Success begets success

What doesn't kill you makes you stronger — Nietzsche

If you have been training for at least three months, you know the fighting arts take discipline. Look at what you are already doing. You have a bad day at work or school and you would like to do nothing more than just stay home and sprawl in front of the tube, but you force yourself to grab your training gear and head out the door to class. Though tired as a three-legged sheepdog, you stay the entire 90 minutes, your uniform sopped with sweat, your muscles shaking like a newborn fawn's. With 15 minutes to go, you catch a hard kick in a training drill, but you stay in there, eat the pain and finish the class.

The dictionary defines discipline as control gained by training. Let's take it a step further and say that discipline strengthens your training and training strengthens your discipline.

Laying a Foundation

Strong discipline must be supported by a strong foundation. In the end, it's all about shedding your old ways, and adopting new ones that put you on a positive course for good health, good fitness and continual progress in your martial art. Here are a few simple tricks to implement into your life that, though gimmicky, work for many people:

- Choose a reasonable immediate goal. You might want to lose 40 pounds, but make your immediate goal five. Write it down on several sticky notes — "I'm burning off five pounds" — and place them where they can be seen every day: refrigerator door, bathroom mirror, car dash, school notebook, and on your desk at work.

- Maintain a training log. In the morning, jot yourself a note in it that reads, "I won't eat anything that compromises my weight, health or training goal." Though you write it every morning, pause for a moment to let the meaning sink in. At night, when you fill in your notebook about your day's eating and training, finish by writing something like, "I feel good about the discipline I had today, and tomorrow I'll be successful again."

- Establish a support system, the best being a workout partner who has the same goals as you. Your non-training friends don't always relate and some even mock you when you eat healthily.

- Choose healthy foods you like. If you crunch on carrot sticks every day and you have never liked them, it's not going to take much to sway you to the dark side. Understand from the get-go that you don't have to eat like a rabbit to eat well and power your body for hard martial arts training.

- Enjoy the process. Don't whine, "Ahh man. One lousy piece of toast. I soooo want two." Instead think, "I'm going to eat this single slice of toast slowly and savor each bite. It's all that I need and want, and it helps me to be leaner and ultimately better in my fighting art." Now, this might sound a little stupid and touchy feely, but it really isn't. The idea is to see the positive in everything you do. The more you eat, train and live your life positively, the better your results and the more pleasure you derive from the process.

- Hang pictures of what you want to look like on your fridge and next to your full-length bedroom mirror. Be realistic. If you stand five feet six inches, don't put a picture of a professional basketball player on your icebox door.

- If your weight gain has occurred over the last couple of years, put up an old photo of yourself when you were lean as an incentive to eat right and train hard. Of course your friends or spouse might look at it, and say, "Wow, you looked good back *then*." If you are easily offended, you might want to keep the photo where only you can see it. Or if such cutting remarks steel your resolve, leave it up.

- Find a saying that clicks with you, such as *nothing tastes as good as thin feels* or *one moment on the lips, forever on the hips*. These things have been around for years but they are still powerful when you ponder their meaning. Yes, that piece of fudge tastes good, as does that milkshake, pizza slice, and 42-ounce beer. The pleasure factor, however, is only momentary, a few minutes at best. You chew or sip it, it dances a jig on your taste buds, and you swallow. Man, was that good! But now it's gone and while the taste lingers, soon that too is gone. Oh, but the calories...they didn't go away. They are deep inside, laughing and mocking you. "Gotcha at a weak moment, didn't we," they taunt in their evil syrupy voices. "Now you'll pay aaaah-ha-ha-ha-ha."

- Stop! Before eating that taste treat, that momentary taste treat, think: "Yes, it will taste good...but only for a few seconds. To burn it off, I'll have to jog for an hour, or kick the bag for 45 minutes. Then after all that work, I won't be closer to my weight loss goal, but only where I was before I ate the momentary taste treat."

- Think in terms of getting through today only. Don't worry about what you ate or how you trained yesterday and don't worry about tomorrow. Think today. "Today I'm going to eat a nutritious breakfast and a low-cal midmorning snack. Lunch will be quality protein and a fruit, and my afternoon snack will be another piece of fruit and a protein bar. Dinner, an energy-producing plate of quality carbs and my workout tonight will be one for the books!" Positive, positive, positive. When you wake up tomorrow, return to the beginning of this paragraph and re-read.

- Idol worship (but within reason. No stalking). Choose a physically fit fighter to admire. This could be the top black belt in your school, a tournament champ, an instructor, Bruce Lee, or Jet Li. Understand that these fighters didn't get to where they are by eating pork rinds and 'tater tarts. They got there by eating and training right. Keep the person in the forefront of your mind to act as a deterrent when temptation comes-a-knockin'. And it always does.

- Okay, you went off your eating regimen and the only workout you have had for a week is thumb reps on your television remote control. It's so easy at this point to say, "Heck with it. This is more fun than watching everything I eat and doing extra bag work." Well, it really isn't more fun. Being healthy, energetic and improving rapidly in your fighting art is far more enjoyable than laziness and gluttony. Okay, maybe for the first week it's a little fun, but by week two or three, when you start feeling sluggish again, moving cow-like and maybe even mooing, you remember why you started on a better nutrition and training program in the first place.

- An occasional relapse is inevitable, but don't use it as an excuse to go off your plan. When it happens, recognize it for what it is and get back on course. Maybe you got hurt, sick or took a two-week vacation. Well, you needed a vacation and getting hurt and sick is part of life. That was then and this is now, so get it in gear and get back at it.

Plan for Problem Periods

Plan right now for the inevitable occasion when you get off track. For example, the chance of you getting a cold is almost an absolute, so think about it now when you are feeling fine and understand that you might be tempted to eat comfort foods. Tell yourself now that it won't happen. Understand and accept that the healthier you eat when sick, the faster you get better. Maybe you are too sick to go to your martial arts school and train, but unless your illness has you totally immobile, you can at least drop down on the floor and do a little light stretching. Eat quality nutrients to make war with the virus and stretch a little to get your blood flowing and loosen your muscles. That is the warrior approach to dealing with illness.

Relapse

For our purposes here, the word relapse means that you have returned to the bad habits you had before your training or diet regimen. Clearly you want to avoid this, but there are times when it's a real test of your will not to slip back into those old patterns. (It's not easy being human). Here are a few tips our students have found helpful to combat this dreaded word:

- Identify situations that might put you at high risk for relapse, such as parties, beer with your buddies, vacation, family commitments, and others. Write them down and ponder ways to avoid them. If you can't or don't want to avoid them, think of how you can get through them without losing everything you have struggled for.

- Write down the consequences of relapsing. Say you have a week long vacation coming up and it's all about sun, fun, and food. Since the rest and relaxation will be good for you physically and mentally, you are allowing for a three-pound weight gain. Is this approach dangerous? A little, especially if you go into it without an understanding of the consequences of going overboard.

- It's helpful to make a list ahead of time of your weaknesses: One Hawaiian drink always leads to three; you always rationalize that it's your vacation so you can eat anything and everything. Then make a list of the consequences of losing control: Since you gained six pounds it will take a month of hard training just to get back to where you were before you went on vacation. Think about your weaknesses and plan how to deal with them before you go. Keep the consequences in the forefront of your mind to act as a buffer when your voice of reason grows feint.

- Before you skip a training session because you are tired, analyze your fatigue to determine if you are simply fooling yourself. If you studied hard all day or slaved over a pile of forms at work, the fatigue you feel, though real, isn't muscle fatigue. It's stress, so a good hard workout is exactly what you need. However, if your job had you hauling giant stones up a hill all day — that is real muscle fatigue and you probably should take a day off from training (and spend the time looking for a new career). Understand that your body often lies to you because it loves your sofa. Always listen to your body's complaints with a critical ear.

- Eliminate all self-talk that tries to justify the good in eating a monster burger and fries and skipping tonight's training session. Understand, that it's not difficult to self-talk your way into or out of things, so make a point that it's always directed at the benefits of eating high-octane food and the importance of consistent training.

- Are you the type of person who jumps into something with both feet and a ton of enthusiasm, but the instant there is a roadblock or a setback, you quit? This is a very real psychological quirk (no it doesn't mean you are crazy or the men in white coats are looking for you) and you should consider seeking counsel from a coach, psychologist or from peers who have overcome it. You need to address the problem because it will affect your martial arts training and dieting efforts.

- Be alert to marketing tricks when shopping for groceries. Know that the super-yummy, calorie-dense, ultra-high fat foods are placed at eye height and in those places that get the most foot traffic. Know that a grocery store is designed to lead you into temptation at every turn. To combat this, always eat before you go shopping and tell yourself ahead of time that you are going to buy only those items on your grocery list. Be strong and don't be manipulated by evil marketing ploys.

- Plan ahead to have healthy snacks available for those rest and relaxation times. When watching the game on Sunday afternoon, be sure to have a sports drink, protein bar and a selection of fruit on hand so you can laugh in the faces of chips and dip, pizza and pop (faces?). Think of yourself as a general preparing for battle. Position your troops (will power, healthy food, positive self-image, goals) in the best position to fight the ever-present enemy (unhealthy treats, temptation, rationalization). Dumb analogy? Maybe. But if it works, use it.

Dealing with Binges

Losing weight or just living a healthy lifestyle takes discipline, a lot of it. But even a Shaolin monk can lose control. For any variety of reasons, any of us can suddenly tear into a plate of goodies like a road vulture on a just-run-over groundhog.

In the past, co-author Demeere has devoured an entire box of chocolate cookies at one sitting (his personal best time was under two minutes) and sloshed it all down with a bottle of a sugar-dense soda pop. These days he binges rarely because he now understands the cause of the problem: It usually happens when he has been following a particularly strict diet without the release of a Dirt Day, especially when sleep deprivation and an exceptionally hard work schedule is added to the mix. He also knows that it takes a lot of extra training to burn off the evil junk food calories.

Christensen knows that his discipline weakens when his family is together for a birthday celebration or a holiday. Though he begins the day with good intentions, when the cake and pizza are laid out, and everyone is gathered around, his will deflates like air from a punctured balloon. Since he knows this about himself, he talks about it - to himself.

A few months before this writing, Christensen lost several pounds and got into top condition to film an instructional martial arts video. Two weeks before the shoot, his family had a birthday party and, knowing his vulnerability, he did a lot of self-talking before the gathering. He told himself that he would have only one piece of pizza and one small slice of cake without ice cream. He talked about how viewers of his tape wouldn't know or even care that he binged on junk food a few days before the shoot, but they would notice his jelly belly. He told himself that he would stay disciplined during the party, linger over each slice and, under no circumstances, would he return for seconds. The self-talk worked! He did exactly what he told himself to do, and he still had a good time with his family. More on self-talk in a moment.

Just as alcoholics have to learn that they can have a good time with friends and family without getting drunk, we too need to accept the fact that we can have a nice time without stuffing ourselves with junk that is harmful to our health and training.

Stack the Deck in Your Favor

Minimize opportunities to binge. If it's your Dirt Day, don't buy extra large portions of candy and other junk food, but buy just one bar of chocolate, one small bag of potato chips or one small portion of ice cream. Get only enough to eat right at that moment; don't take anything home with you. Demeere knows that if chocolate is in the house, he is at risk, so he doesn't buy enough to take home, and Christensen says that because cookies have actually called out to him from the kitchen, he no longer keeps them in the house.

Here is what noted hapkido and self-defense instructor Alain Burrese[38] had to say about a conversation he had with bodybuilder, author and diet expert Clarence Bass. [39]

"Clarence says he will eat anything, fattening things as well. He joked that when he used to take his son out for ice cream he would get caught by people who read his books and columns. He says one key is to not deny yourself totally. He would eat those kinds of things away from home, but keep them out of the house. Using ice cream as an example, he says that it's too easy to eat the whole gallon at home, so he fulfills his cravings by going out for it once in a while. And since he knows he can go out and get it at any time, he never feels deprived."

?

What Pushes Your Binge Button?

√ Fatigue

√ An angry boss

√ The printer ate your work proposal or term paper

√ A parking ticket

√ A bad mood

√ Depression

√ Happiness

√ Eating with family or friends

√ Relationship problems

Emotions and situations are powerful triggers that can lead you down a dark path. If this is you, think about it right now and understand what it is that pushes your "Binge" button. What happens just before that button is poked? How do you justify binging? What thought processes occur when you reach for that third slice of pizza? That fourth? Fifth?

When You Slip

First, don't go getting suicidal on us. Slipping up once in a while just proves you are subject to all the weaknesses of the flesh. It doesn't mean it's hopeless and that you should give up; it does mean that you persevere, just as you do in your training. Although you have some extra calories to burn, learn from the experience and avoid making the same mistake again.

As a veteran personal trainer, Demeere teaches his clients that eating healthily is a long-term plan since short-term ones are destined to fail. If they want only to exercise and diet for as long as it takes to lose weight and then return to their old ways, they are going to put the weight back on. Although this is a simple concept, many of his clients refuse to think long-term. Even when he warns them that short-term thinking makes their goal short lived, some still persist in eating poorly, all the while wanting a rock hard, chiseled physique. Those who keep on training and trying, sooner or later realize that only a long-term strategy, one based on sound nutrition and quality exercise carries them to the goals they want.

Demeere calls this change of thinking "The switch." It's as if the client suddenly flips on a light that illuminates the very truth he has been telling them all along. Many of his new clients, for example, feel that a personal trainer is a short cut to their goals, a person who somehow knows the secret to quick weight loss and optimum health. When Demeere dashes their hopes by telling them there are no such things, some understand, while others need to let it process for a while until they eventually experience The Switch. Once they accept the truth, they begin improving.

Why not make it a goal to be as healthy as possible this date next year, and a long-term goal to be as healthy as possible this date 10 years from now? If you are going to be around anyway, why not be as healthy as you can? Yes, there will be times when you gorge on high-calorie junk food, and times you attack that all-you-can-eat pizza bar so hard you turn a deep shade of green after, but don't worry about it. Fallibility is part of being a humanoid. But being human also means you can correct the slip-up by getting back on course the next day.

Self-talk

There is power in positive self-talk, but before we get to that, be warned that there is also power in negative self-talk. For example, when you continuously tell yourself that...

• dieting is hard

• I will never lose weight

• I'm too tired to train

• I have to feel stuffed after every meal

• losing weight is impossible

• my weight is a result of me being big boned

• being overweight is healthy

• big is beautiful

• I have to eat and drink a lot to be social

...your subconscious begins to believe these things, and when it believes them, it directs your conscious self to do what is necessary to fulfill the perceived truth. Henry Ford must have liked bumper stickers, too, because he said:

"Whether you think you can or whether you think you can't, you're right."

Though Ford's words probably referred to success in the auto industry, they hold true to your efforts at eating healthily and training to be the best you can be. The key to success, and most successful people agree, is to believe that you can attain it. This isn't difficult, but it does take effort: repetition of positive data, careful self-monitoring to block all negative thoughts that try to get in, and fast countering with positive data.

Think of your subconscious as a videotape. Most people fill their tape with negative thoughts: "I can't diet;" "I just love food too much to follow that plan;" "I'll never lose weight;" "I won't get in shape in time for the tournament." Since these negative thoughts have been imprinted deeply into their tape by virtue of repetition, all their conscious actions fulfill their meanings. They find that indeed they can't diet; they love food too much to even try; they never stay on a plan long enough to see results; and they can't get into condition for competition. They haven't a chance for success because their subconscious minds dictate their every conscious, negative move.

Enough! It's time to copy over the tape with powerful, action-filled and success oriented thoughts.

How to Program

Right after the alarm rips you from your slumber, sit up a little so you don't go back to sleep and begin to do the four-count breathing regimen described below. Your mind is calm and receptive to positive self-talk upon awakening, and after three cycles of deep breathing you will be even more so. Here is how you do it. Count to yourself as you do each phase.

Breath in. "One thousand, two thousand, three thousand, four thousand"

Hold it in. "One thousand, two thousand, three thousand, four thousand"

Breath out. "One thousand, two thousand, three thousand, four thousand"

Hold it in. "One thousand, two thousand, three thousand, four thousand"

This is one cycle. Repeat it at least three more times to enjoy a full sense of deep relaxation.

Now you are ready to talk to yourself. Here are three rules for structuring your sentences:

- Be positive. Instead of saying, "I won't go off my diet," say, "I'm staying on my diet." Or, instead of saying, "I won't eat a slice of pie at dinner," say, "I'll eat good, nutritious food at dinner."

- Your subconscious has trouble grasping past and future. Keep all statements in the present. Instead of saying, "I will lose five pounds over the next three weeks," say, "Each day I lose more weight."

- Your subconscious loves powerful descriptive words. Instead of saying,

"I lost half a pound today," say, "Today a half pound of fat melted from my ever slimming body and I feel lighter and gloriously more comfortable." Yes, such words might be an exaggeration and a little corny, but the idea is to charge your subconscious with positive energy.

Here are a few positive statements to get an idea about how to reprogram your subconscious. We know some of these are a little flowery, but your subconscious loves them.

- "I love the fantastic, result-producing eating plan I'm following."

- "I feel awesome all day because I'm sticking to my championship eating plan."

- "It feels incredible losing a little each day."

- "I'm happily slimmer today and I have tons of incredible energy for my training."

- "I love food and I love the wonderful feeling of eating in moderation."

- "My martial arts are improving dramatically because I'm getting into fantastic condition."

When you are back in bed at night, unwinding from your day and feeling the onset of sleep, say these sentences to yourself again. If you fall asleep in the middle of them, it's okay because your subconscious still heard a little and knows what you are doing.

Say them or think them to yourself throughout the day. No, you don't have to sit in a lotus position and burn incense. The idea is to go about your regular activities but keep the positive thoughts in the forefront of your mind. Say them to yourself while driving alone in your car, think them while standing in line at the grocery, doodle them on notepads and spray paint them on the sides of city busses (we're kidding about the busses). It's important to say them and think them often so that they dominate your subconscious to direct your life and goals in a positive direction. [40]

A Powerful Tool that Works

Self-talk has been used successfully in athletics for many years. Super achievers in the sports world as well as those in endeavors outside of it have found it to be a powerful tool that helps them achieve their goals. Some say it was the deciding factor that nudged them from failure to success. It's important to understand that self-talk must be geared towards your needs and your personality. A technique that works for your training buddy might not work for you.

Self-talk doesn't have to be touchy-feely, nor do you have to dance barefoot in a green, sunshine-filled meadow with flowers in your hair while grooving to '60s music. On the other

hand, that might be the very thing that works for you. Most fighters, though, favor a practical, easy-to-apply, hands-on approach. Begin with the techniques described in this chapter and, if you need more information, check out your local bookstore for books, tapes and videos on the subject. Turtle Press offers a wonderful book called *Total MindBody Training* that contains an excellent section on self-talk and psyching up.

The Right Mindset for You

As noted before, just because something works for your teacher or the top black belt in your school, doesn't mean it will for you. Maybe you need a combination of things, ideas that come from multiple sources. If that is the case, so be it. It doesn't mean anything is wrong with you; it just means you have specific needs. Hopefully, the information in this book helps, but should you need even more to get you on the right mental track, don't stop looking until you find a workable combination. It's worth the extra effort to find it.

With nearly 55 years of combined trial and error, your authors have found what works for them. Though we each have the same ultimate objective, our individual personalities and histories have formed our specific approaches. Take a look at what helps us stay on course and if there is anything that you want to borrow, please do. If not, keep on searching.

How Christensen Does It

In the military and law enforcement community, a warrior is often defined as "one who moves toward the sound of guns while everyone else flees" and "one who does what needs to be done." As a soldier in Vietnam, a police officer in a major city and a martial artist since 1965, Christensen has led the life of a warrior. He says that even if he hadn't served in a war, danced the waltz of crooks and cops and trained in the martial arts, he would still be a warrior because warriorhood is a state of mind. It's in this mind-set that he conducts his life.

Christensen believes a warrior should be in top physical and mental condition, that there is no place in warriorhood for a big gut, sluggish moves, and poor discipline. It's this belief that motivates him to push away that big piece of cake and to keep training. When he gains two or three unwanted pounds (usually on vacation), he quickly takes it off since it's incongruous with his self-image. As a warrior teacher, Christensen leads by example, training harder than his students, staying physically fit and encouraging others to do the same.

His self-image keeps his discipline strong when it comes to maintaining his weight and staying in fighting condition. Where most people his age are content to attack buffets, scratch their bellies and sprawl on the sofa, he uses high-power nutrition to keep him going fast and hard. He does this because he likes how it makes him look, feel, perform in the martial arts and — because it's what a warrior does.

How Demeere Does It

Demeere has learned that it isn't one magic bullet that works for him. He requires an integrated approach that employs many big and little things that when combined yield long and lasting results. He has tried numerous diets, fads and gimmicks, finding that they never come close to their grandiose promises. It wasn't that they didn't work at all, but it was that they worked only a little. Through trial and error and lots of persistence, he discovered that when he combined one or more methods, he reached his objective faster. For example, when he combined a healthy nutrition plan with hard training, sufficient rest and knowledge of the idiosyncrasies of his body and mind, his progress took off like a rocket. As a result of this learned self-knowledge, he now approaches whatever diet plan he undertakes with total control, as well as control of all the other support factors.

Demeere knows he has a tendency to gain weight easily. When he stops training and relaxes his diet a little, usually when injured, on holiday or because of work conflicts, the pounds glom onto his hips. Of course it doesn't help that he is an incurable chocolate addict in a land where chocolate reigns supreme. So when his weight increases two or three pounds, he knows he has allowed several factors to get out of control, and he immediately gets back on course. For every half pound of fat that disappears, he is motivated to keep at it, and every pound he loses drives him even harder. Not until he reaches his goal does he relax a little and assume a maintenance regimen.

Learning from Past Problems

Perhaps you have tried several times to get on the right path to a sound nutritional plan, but you have always crashed in flames. Well, welcome to the club. It's easy to make the decision to stay on course for the rest of your life, but sticking to it is hard. Since knowledge is power, look at your previous dieting attempts to determine what went wrong. Were there negative contributing factors that reared up, such as relationship commitments, work schedules and too many party hearty times? How was your motivation going in? Was it a crazy fad diet that drained your energy and motivation, and lead to binging? Did work or school distract you? Did you try to diet during the holidays?

The effort you put into careful and honest analysis of your past efforts helps you avoid those same problems next time. Learn from your mistakes and eventually you will hit on a program that is just right for you.

When You Crash and Burn

Okay, the evil, syrupy voice convinced you to pork out on a monster order of fries and a triple cheeseburger dripping with grease and sauce. Hello guilt! You feel so badly that you seriously consider lifting a garbage dumpster lid and slamming it on your face. While guilt and self-destructive thoughts are human reactions to backsliding, they only make matters worse. Each time you criticize yourself or tell yourself that you can't do this any longer, you reinforce failure and weakness in your subconscious. Do it often enough and those negative tapes you copied over earlier will once again dominate and direct your actions.

Do you see yourself in any of the following situations? If so, read the follow-up comments to help you get back on track:

- **"I binged like a maniac. I'll never be able to eat right!"** Don't view everything related to your behavior as black or white; know that there is a tremendous amount of gray involved. Because you binged at a party one time, doesn't mean you can't get back on track. Don't expect perfection or a flawless record. You are human and therefore allowed to make mistakes. Determine what went wrong and then jump right back into your healthy eating plan.

- **When someone gives you a compliment, you always deny it.** A friend says you look like you lost weight and you come right back with, "Oh, no. I'm so fat. Look at my gut." Don't do that! It programs negativity into your subconscious even more deeply. If getting a compliment is uncomfortable for you, just say, "Thank you. I've been working on it." That keeps it positive.

- **You think: "I'll never lose weight. The heck with this stupid diet,"** because you overdid it at dinner and your pants are ready to burst. Tomorrow you return to your old way of eating with a special emphasis on burgers, pop and chips. At the end of the week you step on the scale and the $@!!$# arrow is pointing four pounds higher than it did last week. You are so depressed you could kick out a stained glass window.

Hey, lighten up a little. You felt stuffed and guilty after hitting the mashed potatoes too hard, so you took a huge mental jump to believing your effort was beyond repair. By overreacting you created a self-fulfilling prophecy that led to a backward slide. That is what is called turning a mosquito into an elephant. The next time it happens, focus on the present: "Okay, I messed up at dinner, but dinner is over." Don't carry the problem any further. Get back into your regimen at breakfast and keep looking toward your goal.

- **Somehow you miscalculated your caloric needs.** You step on the bathroom scale the day before a big tournament and discover you lost only five pounds, but you needed to lose eight to make the weight cat-

egory. So in panic you fast all day and skip breakfast the day of the tournament. You manage to make weight, but when you step into the ring, you feel like stomped on dog doo-doo and your opponent yawns with boredom as he racks up point after point. Defeated, you shake your head and mutter, "I should have known better."

"Should" is a powerful word. It's easy to know the answers *after* they have been given to you, as hindsight is always 20-20. Okay, so you either miscalculated or erred in your plan to lose weight. Don't dwell on what you should have done because that time has already passed. Learn from your mistakes and get on with it.

These are just a few examples of how you can sabotage your efforts of eating properly for your training, recuperation and long-term health. They are the infamous potholes on the road to success. When you drive on a highway and see a road sign that reads *Rough Road Ahead*, you automatically turn up your alertness so you can slow, accelerate, swerve or brake for those rough spots. Your nutrition plan is like that road trip. You must be alert for rough spots and then do what you have to do when they appear so you can keep going. It's not the end of the world when you hit a pothole. Just grip your steering wheel harder and stay in control. But stay alert for the next one; there will be more.

Just as proper nutrition is half the battle in your training strategy, mental commitment — getting your head on right — is half the battle in staying on course. Without it, you are like a car without a steering wheel on that rough road. If you mess up along the way, re-read this chapter and revisit the techniques we suggest. Then start over. Here is another bumper sticker.

Starting over is no big deal, but staying off course is.

Conclusion

Healthy eating and a healthy lifestyle are part of a synergistic approach to becoming the best martial artist you can be. Good nutrition leads to good health, and good health leads to productive training. When you are brimming with health, the world is a more positive and happier place, which makes you a more dynamic person, and the more dynamic you are, the more apt you are to want to learn and get better in whatever martial arts system you enjoy. It's one continuous and ever growing circle.

If you don't make time to eat healthily and exercise,
you must make time to be sick

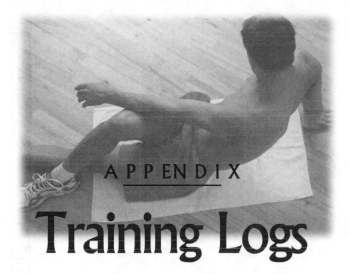

APPENDIX

Training Logs

Use these training logs as presented here or tweak them to fit your likes and particular needs. When you fill them in daily, as we have discussed throughout this book, they become an instant measure as to what you are doing right or where you need to make changes. While taking the time to fill in the logs might seem an annoyance at first, within a week it will be part of your daily routine, one that you will wonder how you ever did without.

Tips

- Photocopy these logs or recreate them to your liking on a spreadsheet program in your computer.

- Fill in the logs in detail or keep them general. They are yours, so use them in whatever way suits your needs.

- Keep them up to date. It's best to fill them in right after your meal or training session when the information is still fresh in your mind. Do it later and you might forget pertinent details, defeating the purpose of the logs.

- Analyze the data once a week, say, Sunday evening. Did you eat too many calories during the past week? Did you do enough heavy bag training? Why did you feel tired on Tuesday? Are you ready to increase your aerobics time? Careful analysis of your logs provides instant answers.

- It's vital that your input is accurate, honest and complete so that it provides information that helps you.

- Know that your eating plan and training regimen are ever changing. Your logs will make that abundantly clear.

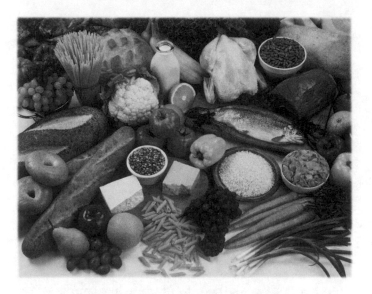

Nutrition

Notice there are columns for your three main meals and three snacks a day. If it has a calorie, it gets noted. Be accurate as you fill these in so you know exactly where to adjust. Be sure to note the time where indicated because knowing when you eat helps you understand your energy levels. You can enter the protein, carbs, fat and calories data into the meals and snacks columns (though it might get crowded), or just enter the day's total in the last one.

Nutrition Log Sample:

Date	Breakfast	Snack	Lunch	Snack	Dinner	Snack	Calories
1/1/	7.30am 2 Eggs, 1/4 cup ham and muffin, no butter Tea	10am Cup yogurt and 1/4 cup all-bran Water	1.30pm 4 oz chicken breast, cup of fruit, mixed bean salad, 1 toast Ice tea	4.30 pm Protein shake	8pm 4 oz chicken, 1 cup of corn, 3/4 cup brown rice, 8 oz milk	10pm Orange juice	Carbs = 1,200 Protein = 680 Fat = 420 Total = 2,300

Date	Breakfast	Snack	Lunch	Snack	Dinner	Snack	Calories

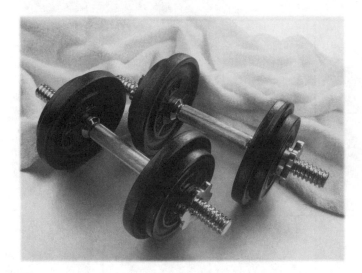

Strength/Cardio

Note the name of each exercise, poundage, reps and rest times in the respective columns, and always comment on how you felt during your session. In the cardio section, note what you did, how long you trained and, if relevant, the distance covered. Include your heart rate, as it is an indicator of your fitness level. The calorie box is for your best guesstimate as to how many were burned during your training. Never skip the comment section, because it's critical when studying past routines.

Strength/Cardio Trainng Log Sample:

Date	Exercise	Set 1 Wt./Rep	Set 2 Wt./Rep	Set 3 Wt./Rep	Set 4 Wt./Rep	Set 5 Wt./Rep	Rest	Comments
1/20	Curls	40/12	50/10	60/8	80/4		1 min.	Good energy

Cardio	Time	Distance	HR	Calories	Comments
Jogging	30	3.5	150	525	Felt good

Date	Exercise	Set 1 Wt./Rep	Set 2 Wt./Rep	Set 3 Wt./Rep	Set 4 Wt./Rep	Set 5 Wt./Rep	Rest	Comments	Cardio	Time	Distance	HR	Calories	Comments

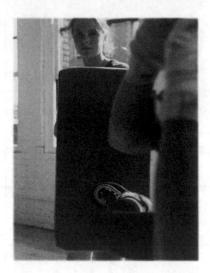

Martial Arts

Use this log to keep track of your progress as you structure and implement various training programs over your career. The four primary components of martial arts training - drills, heavy bag, sparring and forms — are included, with columns large enough for you to note pertinent data in each. Always fill in the comments box.

Martial Arts Trainng Log Sample:

Date	Drills	Time	Heavybag	Time	Sparring	Time	Forms	Time	Other	Time	Comments
18-Jan	Lunge step with backfist 3x10 reps	5	5x3min. rounds of free combinations 1 min. rest between rounds	20	Shadowsparring 5x3min. rounds 1 min. rest between rounds	20	Forms 1 and 2 3 times each	20	Extra stretching during cool-down		Felt tired today

Date	Drills	Time	Heavybag	Time	Sparring	Time	Forms	Time	Other	Time	Comments

References

Chapter 1

1) *Vitaliteit* (Belgium television program) " 3/19/2002

Chapter 2

2) "Jackie Chan interview," *New Line Cinema*, http://www.newline.com/jackiechan/Chan/chaninterview.html

3) Bruce Lee Divine Wind, Interview with Davis Miller, http://www.bruceleedivinewind.com/davis1.html

Chapter 3

4) *Men's Health Guide to Peak Conditioning*, "Carbohydrates," Richard Laliberte, Stephen C. George and editors of Men's Health Books. (1997)

5) *The Science of Martial Arts Training*, Charles I. Staley, published by Unique Publications

6) *Fitness: The Complete Guide*, "Hatfield Estimate for determining daily protein requirements," by Frederick C. Hatfield Ph.D., published by International Sports Sciences Association

7) *Human Kinetics*, "Power eating" by Susan Kleiner with Maggie Greenwood-Robinson (September 2001)

8) *Men's Health Today 2000*, edited by Kenneth Winston Caine, Men's Health Books, Rodale, Inc, St. Martin's Press. (2000)

9) *Muscle & Fitness Online*, "Basic Strategies for Getting Lean," by Dave Picard, http://www.muscleandfitness.com/nutritionsupp/p/2785.jsp.

10) "Women and Midlife Weight Gain - The Battle of the Bulge!", by Jana Klaure MD, http://partnership.hs.columbia.edu/klauer.html

Chapter 4

11) *Carbohydrate Loading*, "Carbohydrates in Nutrition" by Ron Kenedy MD., http://www.medical-library.net/sites/carbohydrates_in_nutrition.html

12) *Carbohydrate loading*, "Con in the "carbo-loading argument," by L. Lee Coyne, Ph.D, http://www.centralhome.com/ballroomcountry/carbohydrate-loading.htm

13) *Inside Kung Fu*, 1/1/01, "Frank Shamrock's Ultimate Training and Fighting System" by John Steven Soet

Chapter 5

14) *Nutrition for serious athletes*, by Dan Bernardot PhD, published by Human Kinetics

15) Gennari, C. & Nuti, R. (1998). Other agents for the treatment of osteoporosis. In *Osteoporosis: Diagnosis and Management* (P. Meunier, ed.). London: Martin Dunitz.

16) Avioli, L. V. (1993). Calcium and bone: Myths, facts and controversies. In *The Osteoporotic Syndrome: Detection, Prevention and Treatment*, 3rd ed. (Avioli, ed.). New York: Wiley-Liss.

17) *The Physician and Sports Medicine*, "Minding Your Minerals: Iron, Zinc, Selenium, and Chromium," Nancy Clark, MS, RD - VOL 24 - NO. 6 - (JUNE 1996)

18) *Runner's World*, "Dig These Minerals," October 1995, by Liz Applegate, Ph.D.

19) *Nutrition for serious athletes*, by Dan Bernardot PhD, published by Human Kinetics

20) *Facts About Dietary Supplements*, by the National Institutes of Health Clinical Center http://www.cc.nih.gov/ccc/supplements/iron.html

Chapter 6

21) *Hydrate*, Muscle Media, Spring

22) *Canadian Journal of Applied Physiology*, "Caffeine and Neuromuscular Fatigue in Endurance Athletes," Vol. 19, Supplement, 1994, and "Comparison of Coffee and Caffeine as an Ergogenic Aid," Canadian Journal of Applied Physiology, Vol. 19, Supplement,1994

23) Urban Legends reference page; http://www.snopes.com/toxins/water.htm

Chapter 7

24) "Mark Dacascos Chat," *Mystique's Mad Realm*, http://www.markdacascos.org

25) "Talking Tae-Bo: An Interview with Billy Blanks," by Amazon.com's Special Interests editor, Jenny Brown, http://www.amazon.com

26) "Frank Shamrock's Ultimate Training and Fighting System" or Inside Kung Fu by John Steven Soet 1/1/01

Chapter 9

27) *The Science of Martial Arts Training*, Charles I. Staley, published by Unique Publications

28) *Dr. Squat*, "The Zigzag diet , Frederick C. Hatfield, .www.drsquat.com

Chapter 10

29) *British Medical Journal*, "Frequency of eating and concentrations of serum cholesterol in the Norfolk population of the European prospective investigation into cancer," Bingham S, Welch A, et al. (2001)

Chapter 11

30) *Health Guide to Peak Conditioning*, "Creatine," Richard Laliberte, Stephen C. George and editors of Men's Health Books. Rodale Press, Inc, Emmaus, Pennsylvania, (1997)

31) *Medicine and Science in Sports and Exercise*, "Effect of creatine loading on long-term sprint exercise performance and metabolism," Preen, D., Dawson, B., Goodman, C., Lawrence, S., & Beilby, J. (2001).

32) From an interview with Daniella Somers by co-author Wim Demeere.

Chapter 12

33) *Science of Martial Arts Training*, by Charles I. Staley, published by Unique Publications

34) *Fitness: The Complete Guide*, by Frederick C. Hatfield, published by International Sports Sciences Association

35) *Science of Martial Arts Training*, by Charles I. Staley, published by Unique Publications

Chapter 13

36) *IronMag.com*, unknown author http://www.ironmag.com/ct_knowledge_05.html

37) *Run Quick*, "The five iron laws of quick running," unknown author, http://www.runquick.com/corcorn/5laws.htm

Chapter 14

38) Alain Burrese is a popular author and martial arts instructor. Visit him on his web site at http://www.burrese.com

39) Clarence Bass's is a long-time bodybuilder and popular author on the topic of sensible training and dieting. Visit him on his website at http://www.cbass.com

40) *The Mental Edge, Revised*, by Loren W. Christensen, Desert Publications, (1999)

Website Sources

www.turtlepress.com: Turtle Press website

www.lwcbooks.com : co-author Loren W. Christensen's website

www.grindingshop.com : co-author Wim Demeere's website

www.gella.be Gella Vandecaveye's website, judo world champion

www.daniellasomers.com Daniella Somers's website, boxing and kickboxing world champion

www.modernfighter.com Martina Sprague's website, author and kickboxer

www.myodynamics.com Charles I. Staley's, website, martial arts and strength training specialist

www.drsquat.com, Frederick C. Hatfield's website, strength training expert

Books Referenced, Mentioned and Recommended

* *Warrior Speed* by Ted Weimann, published by Turtle Press

* *Speed Training: How to develop your maximum speed for martial arts*, by Loren W. Christensen, published by Paladin Press

* *The Mental Edge, Revised,* by Loren W. Christensen, Desert Publications

* *Total MindBody Training: A guide to peak athletic performance*, by Jacob H., M.D. Jordan, published by Turtle Press

* *Fighter's Fact Book: Over 400 concepts, principles and drills to make you a better fighter*, by Loren W. Christensen, published by Turtle Press

* *Solo Training: The martial artist's guide to training alone*, by Loren W. Christensen, published by Turtle Press

" *Fighting Power: How to develop explosive punches, kicks, blocks and grappling*, by Loren W. Christensen, published by Paladin Press

* *Dynamic Tension*, by Harry Wong, published by Unique Publications

* *Science of Martial Arts Training* by Charles I. Staley MSS, published by Unique Publications

* *Periodization: Theory and Methodology of Training* by Tudor O. Bompa, PhD., published by Human Kinetics Pub.

Index

fast-twitch muscle fibers 192–196
fat 20, 24, 42, 56–57, 61, 66, 73–78,
    136, 140, 149, 170
fat-free 29
fat-soluble vitamins 56, 74, 84, 87
fatigue 253
flexibility 241
folic acid 87
food intolerance 222
fortified 84, 89
foundation-eating plan 118, 120
free-hand exercises 192–205
front kick 179

G

glucose 66–68, 70, 78, 105, 110–111
Glycemic Index 45–46, 219–221
glycogen 67–71, 111
goal 186, 233, 250
good eating habits 80
grappling 195
green tea 113–114

H

hardening exercises 241
Hatfield Estimate 51–54, 60
HDL cholesterol 95, 109
health 229–230
health food 18, 27
heart disease 78
heavy bag 143–146, 156
Hell Week 170
herbal weight-loss products 26–30
high blood pressure 113
high cholesterol 76
high impact training 149
High Intensity Interval Training 136, 139–
    146, 173
high-fat diet 76
high-protein diet 77
HIIT 136, 139–146, 173
hunger 171
hyperglycemia 70
hyperthermia 101
hyponatremia 106
hypothermia 101

I

ideal weight 160, 163
Infomercials 31–32
injuries 150, 231–232, 238–243
insulin 70, 73
International Olympic Committee 111
iron 96

J

jump kicks 178
junk food 131, 162

K

kickboxing. 148
kicking 136, 156, 199, 177–182
kneeling kicking drill 179

L

labels 27, 29
lactase 115
lactose intolerant 115
laxatives 167
LDL cholesterol 57, 78, 95
lean body mass 51
lifestyle changes 169
liquid diets 66, 80
liquids 98
low carb/high protein diets 66
low fat 28–30, 66, 116
low-carb diet 68–70
lunch 124

M

machine gun kicks 156, 178
macrocycle 228, 233–238
macrominerals 95
macronutrients 44
magnesium 93
making weight 159–166
Maximum Heart Rate 184
meals 23, 168, 171, 223
medical check up 243
menopause 93
menstrual cycle 96
mesocycle 236–237
mesomorph 34, 37–39
metabolism 22, 61, 62, 163, 168
microcycle 237–238

About The Authors

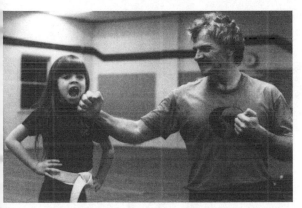

Loren Christensen with his youngest daughter Amy

Loren W. Christensen began studying the martial arts in 1965. Over the years he has earned 10 black belts, seven in karate, two in jujitsu and one in arnis. He used his training as a military policeman in Saigon, Vietnam, a police officer for 25 years in Portland, Oregon, and as a karate tournament competitor, capturing 53 wins.

As a free-lance writer, Loren has authored 25 books (half of them on the martial arts), dozens of magazine articles and edited a newspaper for nearly eight years. He has recently starred in five instructional martial arts videos.

Retired from police work, Loren now writes full time, teaches martial arts to a small group of students, and gives seminars on the martial arts, police defensive tactics, and verbal judo. To contact Loren, visit his website LWC Books at www.lwcbooks.com.

Wim Demeere began training at the age of 14, studying the grappling arts of judo and jujitsu for several years before turning to the kick/punch arts of traditional kung fu and full-contact fighting. Over the years he has studied a broad range of other fighting styles, including muay Thai, kali, pentjak silat and shootfighting. Since the late 1990s, he has been studying tai chi chuan and its martial applications.

Wim's competitive years saw him win four national titles and a bronze medal at the 1995 World Wushu Championships. In 2001, he became the national coach of the Belgian Wushu fighting team.

A full-time personal trainer in his native country of Belgium, Wim instructs both business executives and athletes in nutrition, strength and endurance, and a variety of martial arts styles. He has managed a corporate wellness center and regularly gives lectures and workshops in the corporate world. You can contact Wim through his website The Grinding Shop at www.grindingshop.com

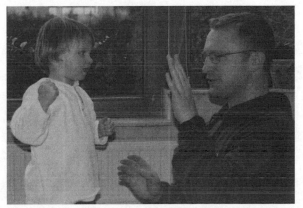

Wim Demeere with his daughter Lauren

Also Available from Turtle Press:

The Science of Takedowns, Throws and Grappling for Self-
defense
Fighting Science
Martial Arts Instructor's Desk Reference
Guide to Martial Arts Injury Care and Prevention
Solo Training
Fighter's Fact Book
Conceptual Self-defense
Martial Arts After 40
Warrior Speed
The Martial Arts Training Diary
The Martial Arts Training Diary for Kids
TeachingMartial Arts
Combat Strategy
The Art of Harmony
Total MindBody Training
1,001 Ways to Motivate Yourself and Others
Ultimate Fitness through Martial Arts
Weight Training for Martial Artists
A Part of the Ribbon: A Time Travel Adventure
Herding the Ox
Neng Da: Super Punches
Taekwondo Kyorugi: Olympic Style Sparring
Martial Arts for Women
Parents' Guide to Martial Arts
Strike Like Lightning: Meditations on Nature
Everyday Warriors

For more information:
Turtle Press
PO Box 290206
Wethersfield CT 06129-206
1-800-77-TURTL
e-mail: sales@turtlepress.com

http://www.turtlepress.com